What Long-Term Care Leaders are Saying about *Brush Fire*

What really happened in nursing homes during the COVID-19 pandemic? Deke Cateau gives an up close and transparent look in *Brush Fire*. This book mimics Deke's open and honest leadership style, and it gives the reader a glimpse of how difficult this time was for not only the residents who lived in the A.G. Rhodes homes but also for the dedicated and caring staff. The complexities that nursing homes faced are highlighted and explained in this book, coming from the lens of someone with direct experience. What is most impressive, though, is that the person-centered culture of A.G. Rhodes was steadfast during this time. Residents and staff members came first, no excuses, no exceptions. You can't read Deke's book without realizing that nursing homes should not be vilified for how they reacted during the pandemic. They should be honored with the highest praise!

—Penny Cook, MSW
President and CEO, Pioneer Network

Brush Fire is both tragic and encouraging. Through the lens of the 2020 COVID pandemic experience, Deke Cateau brings the story of those working and living in long-term care settings into the bright light of day, including the unbelievable challenges, the moments of hope, and the future potential. I am inspired by how the A.G. Rhodes communities value deep relationships and systems of care focused on care partnerships and visionary leadership practices, and how those can make a significant difference, especially during tough times.

—*Denise Hyde,*
Community Builder, The Eden Alternative®

During the COVID-19 pandemic, most of what you heard in the news was from people with no real perspective on life in long-term care or the challenges operators face delivering service just in normal times. *Brush Fire* is written by someone who knows and lives in the industry. The book focuses on the issues around the pandemic but also gives the reader a real look inside a nursing home which is, as Deke says, both business and a social service. Only good can come from better understanding of long-term care, the challenges and culture change which can shape the future.

—*Andy Isakson*
Managing partner, Isakson Living

The heroic struggle of nursing home leaders during the COVID-19 crisis is epitomized in the stellar example set by Deke Cateau as he fought against horrifying odds to keep the frail and highly vulnerable residents in his care safe, and to keep his staff willing to show up to work, day after day, month after month. SARS-COV-2 is not only a silent and deadly killer of frail older adults—the virus has also laid bare the fundamental flaws in the way we value our elders and provide care for them. Deke and his team of caring warriors have not just battled COVID-19—they have also been subject to misinformed and demoralizing criticism and vilification from policy makers, advocates, and the news media. This needs to change—and Deke Cateau shows the way. Read this book—and then use Deke's big-hearted wisdom to take action!

—*Christopher E. Laxton, CAE*
Executive Director, AMDA—The Society for Post-
Acute and Long-Term Care Medicine

Deke Cateau's professional leadership at A.G. Rhodes and throughout the long-term care industry is quite evident in his book: *Brush Fire: COVID-19 and Our Nursing Homes*. Deke's foresight on social-emotional, psychological, and physical well-being of all residents, staff, and frontline workers and his understanding of the aging boomer population fuels his understanding of the drastic changes that the nursing home industry must undertake to remain a viable care option in the coming years. This book is a must-read for all industry leaders!

—Jackie Pinkowitz, MED
Board Chair, Dementia Action Alliance

With absolute transparency, Deke Cateau shares an unflinching look at the pandemic experience in three Georgia nursing homes. In doing so, he reveals the shortcomings of our nation's elder care system and the courage of those who work in elder care—and he shows us what true leadership is all about.

—G. Allen Power, MD
Geriatrician, Author of Dementia Beyond Drugs

Deke Cateau has chronicled the life of a nursing home during COVID-19 with passion and clarity. His deep commitment to the dignity and quality of life of those he serves, and his complete embrace of person-directed care and service, are exemplary. As Deke so aptly describes, nursing homes play a unique and critical role in our health-care system; there is no excuse for anything short of excellence. All whose life or work touches nursing home care will learn from Deke's leadership. We must, as a country, embrace his action plan for change.

—Katie Smith Sloan
President and CEO, Leading Age

Deke Cateau's honest and self-revealing *Brush Fire* provides readers a view of COVID-19 from the inside—the lived experience of a professional caught at the epicenter of the pandemic—a nursing home. His chapter on residents living with dementia shines a light on the special actions necessary to protect this group—the most vulnerable members of A.G. Rhodes communities.

—*John Zeisel PhD, Hon DSc*
Author: I'm Still Here, *Founder: Hearthstone*
Institute & I'm Still Here Foundation

Contents

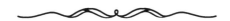

Note about Language from the Author

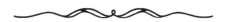

To be clear, language matters! As someone who has been involved in the culture change movement for the last several years, I've been very careful in my use of nomenclature related to the nursing home industry. This book, however, is intended for all readers, especially those who may not know or who may have misconceptions about our industry. For these reasons, I have combined industry language as it's used operationally with usage that the average person recognizes. For example, "facilities" is interchangeable with "communities." In the culture change movement, we tend to avoid the F word, but the term is sometimes used throughout these chapters because not all facilities operate as communities, at least not yet. Similarly, "residents," "elders," and "patients" are used interchangeably. I suspect these and other industry words and definitions will be subject to revision over time. After all, as aging takes on new meaning to different people, so too will the nursing home industry.

Deke Cateau

Foreword

The American long-term care system, particularly in nursing homes, has been exposed by the COVID-19 pandemic as deeply flawed, chronically underfunded, and in need of reform. The sector is in a historic moment, presenting both an immense challenge—and a huge opportunity—to improve outcomes and quality of life for over a million nursing home residents and more than a million frontline workers who care for them every day, as well as millions more who live and work in seniors housing communities nationwide.

This book sheds light on the type of vision and leadership that America's seniors housing and care operators, investors, and partners will need if they are to succeed in the post COVID world. Originally, the promise of senior living was about lifestyle and connectedness. Over the years, however, as owners and operators have sought to meet shifting demands, the sector has followed a trend of rising frailty or acuity levels of its residents. As Americans grow older, larger numbers of seniors require increasing levels of assistance with activities of daily living, such as feeding and dressing. As a result, many senior living operators gradually shifted their focus to marketing care to meet needs rather than offering a lifestyle to provide human connections and a sense of belonging and purpose.

Today, there are more than three million people on any given day whose home is a senior living setting, a number that will grow significantly in coming years. Skilled nursing and assisted living residents average eighty-five-plus years, have multiple chronic conditions, and require assistance with several activities of daily living (ADLs). Significant numbers of these residents also have cognitive impairment. The vast majority require close contact with caregivers day and night. Despite these mobility and cognitive challenges, these older adults want out of their daily life what everyone else wants—something that reaffirms their identity and their sense of self-worth and connectedness to others.

Huge numbers of baby boomers, who will need care and services, will force the system to change. Aside from their sheer numbers, the biggest change will be driven by the collapse in unpaid or informal caregivers, such as spouses and adult children. In years past, the forty-five-to sixty-four-year-old cohort used to bear much of the burden of caring for their elders, but boomers had fewer children than previous generations and those that did have are less likely to live nearby. They also have higher divorce rates. In fact, due to numerous major demographic shifts, the ratio of unpaid caregivers aged forty-five to sixty-four to eighty-plus years old in the US is plummeting. In 2010, that ratio was seven to one. In 2030, it will drop to four to one. By 2050, it will be three to one. Many of those potential caregivers will not live in proximity to their parents.

Recently, the oldest baby boomer turned seventy-five. A decade from now, this huge and disruptive generation will start to enter the market in large numbers. But they are unlikely to buy today's care-focused products. For many boomers, the experience of COVID has led to a desire not to end up quarantined in a room when they are older.

We're seeing a rejection from tomorrow's customers of today's products. Boomer women who have spent a lifetime fighting to get into the workplace, fighting for their rights, and for independence will not accept a deficit-driven model of aging services that treats them like toddlers or infants. Too many current senior living models reinforce a sense of dependency and helplessness among residents that denies them a sense of independent agency and self-worth. That's contradictory to boomer culture.]

Some industry leaders are already acting to accommodate not only the desires of a new type of customer in the boomers, but to implement a new vision for what it means to provide care and services for our oldest Americans. Under Deke Cateau's leadership and vision, A.G. Rhodes is positioning itself to do much more than survive the COVID-19 pandemic. This organization has managed to provide top quality care for underserved populations for well over a century and has continued to innovate in ways usually associated with private pay consumer environments but for a majority Medicaid clientele. COVID-19 has shown their ability to do this even in the most difficult of times. Deke understands that the task of leaders in a crisis like the COVID-19 pandemic is to manage the crisis while building the future. During this time of disruption, Deke's vision for the future will change the lives of residents and staff for the better while reaping the benefits of a new normal that is in the process right now of becoming a reality.

For too many years, we've had an overemphasis on a care model for seniors that focuses on simply surviving. Now, as Deke clearly sees, we're moving from a care model to a community model that focuses on thriving through engagement. This is not so much a longevity revolution as a vitality revolution, focusing on feeling and being vital and connected to people and places both inside and outside the walls of the home itself. Already many are experimenting with new products that follow boomers through their seventies and into their eighties. Focusing on the values that matter to boomers, such as engagement, connection, and enrichment, these models reflect some of the ideas that you'll find in this book.

What boomers will want is not just amenities or good food but customized personalized experiences tailored to their interests. Boomers have already shown us that they won't buy something they don't think they need. Whatever your passion—whether for grandkids, social change, travel, mentorship, ongoing learning, Italian food, or the arts, whatever—you can be matched through technologies leveraging advanced algorithms and artificial intelligence with other like-minded people. Long before you move to senior living, you can be connected to that affinity group. When and if you do move in, you'll be moving to a place where you can share experiences with a preexisting network of friends.

While I'm bullish on the opportunity to rethink and reimagine senior living and senior care that exists in this moment, I am bearish on whether many current operators will be able to pivot to meet these needs and deliver what future customers will want and need.

For many operators, the struggles with COVID have been painful and expensive. Residents and staff have died. Expenses have far exceeded revenues. Finances are exhausted, and so are the staff. It's a tough time to face such swift and demanding disruption. As a result, we see many new players from other fields moving into the market. Huge tech firms, such as Google and Amazon and Apple, and big retailers, such as CVS, Walmart, and Best Buy, are already carving inroads to take ownership of what they see as a huge potential market, especially enabling people to receive care in the setting they call home. As is the case in any disruption, many new models will fail, either because they don't really understand what will move their customer or they won't be able to scale fast enough. But some will succeed and by doing so, will forever change how we deliver care and services appropriate to the needs of our seniors.

Another disruption will be in the branding of senior living. Successful brands won't even be called senior living. To many boomers, that represents their parents' notion of aging and retirement, and they want nothing to do with it. New models will need to be metaphors for being alive, not places to disappear and die. They will offer places and experiences that lift the spirit and connect residents with experiences that give them joy and a sense of meaning and belonging. As Lisa Marsh Ryerson, president of the AARP Foundation, said in her NIC Talk, "The senior care sector needs to rethink and reposition its activities directors. Instead," she argues, "they should be purpose matchmakers." In her vision, the primary role of these purpose matchmakers is to help that resident find his or her sense of purpose that offers a sense of belonging and connectedness. That won't be bingo every day. Boomers don't want that and will reject it. Again, there's recognition that despite enormous demand, the customers of tomorrow will reject the product of today.

Older adults can and want to be contributors to their communities, not just receivers or takers. There is a community in Washington, DC, that realized that their staff's kids were struggling with virtual learning and that this was a real burden for staff members. The residents adopted several of their kids for mentoring. In Dallas, residents are mentoring foster kids who have suffered the worst as the pandemic shut down their schools. These are just a few examples of what is happening in senior living, especially as retirement as we know it is rethought and redefined as a time to refire, reboot, and regenerate rather than to decline and disappear.

Older adults have something to offer, even as they grow frailer. The Japanese have a great expression, "*Ikigai*," which can be translated as "reason to get up for breakfast." Every person needs that, no matter their age or degree of cognitive or mobility challenges. As Jill Vitale-Aussem has observed in her book, *Disrupting the Status Quo of Senior Living: A Mind Shift*, too often, operators of senior living communities fail to ask the most important questions of their residents. We ask about their underlying health conditions, their difficulty in performing activities of daily living, the drugs they take, and their finances, but we fail to ask the questions that speak to their unique identity and what gives them a sense of belonging and self-worth. Questions such as what gifts, passions, and talents will you bring to this community? What's next for you? Where and how would you like to grow or learn? What do you hope to accomplish in your time living with us? These sorts of questions reframe the focus from what residents have lost and rather speak to what they have and what they hope to do or to accomplish in their months and years ahead. Ultimately, the new customer may be retired in the sense that they no longer work for a living, and they may indeed have a number of mobility or cognitive challenges but very few will wish to be retired from living a fulfilling life.

This is a disruptive moment, not only for nursing home and senior housing operators, but for the US health care system. Payers and providers of health care are realizing that it's essential to move from a health delivery system built around reactive sick care to one based on prevention and proactive management of underlying health conditions. The future, therefore, of promoting health and providing health care services to our growing older population will be delivering services where they live, managing chronic conditions on site through monitoring, and triaging at home whenever possible to prevent unnecessary trips to the emergency department.

COVID-19 has accelerated us into the twenty-first century. The pandemic has swiftly made telemedicine a broadly accepted and funded means to monitor and, in many cases, care for residents on site. This is enabling nursing homes and even seniors housing communities to improve access to health care services without having to expose residents to the risks inherent in a trip to the doctor's office or hospital. Using similar technology, residents can feel connected to the world and can engage in activities with friends and loved ones even when they can't leave their rooms.

Telehealth, while essential, will only be a part of the health care picture in nursing homes and senior living in the future. Operators will need health care providers and payers to help them think through how best to design and deliver packages with options, such as Medicare Advantage plans and managed Medicaid, as health and health care services inevitably become integrated into seniors housing and care settings. Operators will need health care partners in order to provide integrated service delivery onsite.

Again, Deke's leadership and vision are already moving in this direction and have been doing so since before the pandemic hit. His association with the Eden Alternative®—with its focus on combating loneliness, boredom, and helplessness among older adults in senior care settings, which you will read about in this book—is a strong, progressive move in a direction which is not only right for Deke and his team and residents, but for the survival and advancement of his business in coming years. Succeeding in a time of disruption will take vision, but, perhaps most importantly, for leaders in the seniors housing and care industry, it will take a strong culture built on transparency and trust.

This book provides a glimpse into the kind of culture that will succeed—a collaborative team-based culture in which staff and residents are all one family. The key to that commitment is trust. Trust is built upon the foundation of transparent, open, frequent, personal, credible communication with staff and with residents and their families. Of course, Deke's staff understands that he isn't a miracle worker, but they know that he's got their back. He gets the issues that weigh down staff and understands that they are the first people he should consult when trying to do better. During this period of immense disruption, that orientation to frontline staff will make all the difference, as will Deke's ability to envision a new way of delivering care and value to residents, their families, and his staff as well.

Numerous reporters and commentators recently have speculated and some have predicted that fear of congregate living settings due to the pandemic will mean the demise of senior living. To the contrary, months of forced isolation and virtual relationships have made all of us, regardless of age, long for the real thing—human touch, human connection, face-to-face conversation, and relationships and activities that provide a sense of belonging and purpose. For that reason, senior living settings will not disappear, but they will have to change dramatically so that they become aspirational settings and not settings to avoid if you possibly can.

In addition, many have also predicted that this will be the end of nursing homes. However, for those with significant mobility and/or cognitive challenges, the cost on unpaid family caregivers and for paid professional caregivers of providing care in traditional residential homes or apartments can and will be prohibitive. The need for nursing homes will not go away, but, once again, we cannot accept what today we offer as care in nursing homes. We can and must do better and this means radically rethinking how we provide care and how we deliver quality of life for residents and staff. That will require a bold vision and bold leadership. Read on to learn about Deke Cateau's vision for that future and the lessons he's learned through the pandemic.

Robert Kramer
President and founder Nexus Insights,
Cofounder and strategic advisor at the National Investment
Center for Seniors Housing and Care (NIC)

Preface

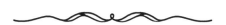

I am, first and foremost, a nursing home administrator. This is the professional accomplishment for which I am most proud. It takes a certain degree of insanity to be as passionate as I am about operating in an industry that is so flawed and carries so many stigmas. I am guilty as charged!

It is safe to say that like most nursing home administrators, I have seen a lot. Like many, I have posited for years that I have seen enough to write a book. Well, here's my shot!

I became an administrator in 2004 at a nursing home in metro Atlanta, where a resident tried to climb out of his second-floor window by tying sheets to the bed frame to use as a rope. Sadly, he fell and died. In another instance, I was called to the nursing home one Saturday morning because a resident tied a noose around another resident's neck and tried to hang him. Luckily, he did not succeed. More recently, a family member came to my nursing home—gun brandishing—because he thought we hurt his mother. I can go on and on.

I've experienced a lot in this industry, but never anything as challenging as COVID-19. It started suddenly and quickly turned into a never-ending nightmare. Month after month, the crisis weighed on us emotionally and physically, and there were no real signs of abating. The rigors of this pandemic rested on our backs, getting heavier and heavier each month. It seemed we bore a cross without hopes of resurrection; vilified by many with absolutely no reprieve. We were in a war with no formal training, no armory, and few weapons. Our battlefield offered few protections. With no hills or gullies to hide in and no time to make sandbags, we were exposed, naked to the elements and illness.

Nothing could have prepared us for the invisible enemy that lurked on every corner as it doubled, tripled, and quadrupled its impact. This foe did not sleep; it just kept steadily advancing. Then it learned to mutate and grow faster and stronger, perfecting its viral craft while being impossible to detect in time to stop it. Its favorite prey was in nursing homes. We were unable to run or hide, left as sitting ducks. We had no choice but to bunker down with imperfect plans and no real exit strategy.

To be fair, the effects of COVID-19 on congregate environments like ours should not have surprised anyone. Most of our residents share rooms, and life in nursing homes consists of group activities and events which facilitate the spread of any infectious disease. We know this because, for decades, we've struggled with other viruses such as the flu, which has caused significant sickness and even death. Nursing homes are also complicated operating units—change in any one department usually has significant ripple effects on other departments and ultimately, considerable impact on our residents' daily lives.

So I understand how this happened, but I'm amazed—and seriously concerned—at the overt vilification and blame placed on the nursing home industry. We are far from perfect, and we have significant issues to address, but we have been unfairly targeted. Through this book, I hope to tell the nursing home industry's side of the story and share firsthand experiences from A.G. Rhodes, a nonprofit nursing home organization with three communities in metro Atlanta. I've had the great honor of working in various positions at A.G. Rhodes for more than a decade, including in my current position as chief executive officer since 2018.

Often in crises, we struggle to see a bigger picture. It's easy for us to see a situation through a narrow lens, but if we widen our lens and open our hearts and minds, we will see a much larger and more complete view. We can make more informed judgements instead of pointing fingers. My hope is that this book will give readers a better viewpoint of nursing home operations. My intent is not to be defensive or judgmental, but to give more context to the cards we've been dealt. Most importantly, this book promotes the need for drastic infrastructural, regulatory, and operational changes in our industry.

Many of the concerns and observations I include in this book have been in my thoughts for years. Quite simply, I did not have the courage or opportunity to express them, but the impact of COVID-19 has emboldened me. It has given me the voice I didn't know I had. More importantly, it has given me clarity in my conviction about what needs to happen. My greatest hope is to encourage others who are involved in the nursing home industry to join me in this conviction. If we focus our collective efforts and use the lessons we've learned throughout this pandemic, we can create transformative reforms and meaningful change to avoid another crisis like COVID-19. Nursing home residents have suffered enough because of this pandemic, and we must come together to do more to protect and care for them.

If you work in a nursing home, please know that this book is not meant to critique you in any way. It's quite the opposite. This book highlights your selflessness and the sacrifices you make each day as you protect our beloved seniors amidst extraordinary and unique challenges. In this spirit, this book is dedicated to those on the nursing home frontlines: the certified nursing assistants, licensed practical nurses, registered nurses, custodial staff, dietary staff, therapists, administrators, support staff, and all who toil day in and day out in our nation's nursing homes. You are indeed our essential workers, our first responders. I salute you!

Chapter 1

$$\sim\!\!\diamond\!\!\sim$$

Ignite

How did we get here?

On February 28, 2020, I woke up in a hotel room in Charlotte, North Carolina. I was there to visit a state-of-the-art Continuing Care Retirement Community (CCRC) also known as a Life Plan Community (LPC). On the news that morning, I saw that some of the first COVID-19 cases reported in the United States emerged in a Washington state nursing home. My heart dropped. I instinctively knew that our lives in this industry would be changed forever. I knew that the conditions in most of our nation's nursing homes would serve as an incendiary to the spread of COVID. Within a matter of days, 129 cases became associated with that nursing home, including eighty-one residents, thirty-four staff members, and fourteen visitors; twenty-three people died.

The community I was visiting in Charlotte was named Aldersgate. It was a beautiful community with three levels of care, including independent living, assisted living, and skilled nursing, which is commonly known as nursing home care. A fantastic and expansive community sitting on 180 acres of attractive Carolina real estate, Aldersgate was a wonderful showpiece of what retirement living should be like. Not the highest end or most glamorous of communities, but extremely charming and elegant and most importantly, homelike. I was there with a team from Georgia to look at design elements we were considering for a new construction project at A.G. Rhodes.

I came to Charlotte a day earlier than our tour because as an added treat, my predecessor at A.G. Rhodes—Al Blackwelder, a mentor and a good friend—recently retired there with his wife, Cyndi. They now own a beautiful cottage home on the outskirts of the Aldersgate campus. Al and I went to dinner the night before the tour along with two leadership staff from Undine, a senior living culinary company that ran the dining operations at both Aldersgate and A.G. Rhodes.

Aldersgate's nursing center, Asbury Health and Rehab, is a perfect example of what every nursing home resident in this country deserves: private room accommodations and beautiful living and dining spaces. The community is set up in neighborhoods of twelve residents and those residents dine together in a small, natural family-like setting, just as most of us do in our own homes. Unlike Aldersgate, the A.G. Rhodes communities are more traditional nursing homes that were built on a medical model of care.

Nursing home origins

Our homes, and most of the 15,000-plus nursing homes across the nation, owe our complicated history to a legacy of asylums, poor houses, and almshouses. Care for residents was largely free with many contributing to their own expenses by working or growing food for their subsistence. A "new" old-age home was established in the early nineteenth century as an alternative, and the quality and oversight of these institutions was greatly improved when the federal government first became involved in nursing homes with the passage of the Social Security Act of 1935. However, care remained institutional and substandard (*Long-Term Care in an Aging Society*, Rowles and Teaser. Springer pub. 2016).

In 1954, amended legislation in the Hill Burton Act provided states with matching federal funds to erect nursing homes in conjunction with hospitals, which resulted in the hospital-like design of most nursing homes today. In 1959, the industry was further stimulated through federal mortgage insurance allowing low-interest loans from private lenders. These measures led to a significant increase in nursing home construction (Committee on Nursing Home Regulation, 1986).

The Nursing Home Reform Act, which was part of the Omnibus Reconciliation Act of 1987 (OBRA '87), resulted in broad base changes and set quality standards within nursing homes across the country. Three decades later, we have seen vast improvements in quality of care and services in our nation's nursing homes, and we continue to improve despite our environmental design.

A. G. Rhodes

A.G. Rhodes was one of the first nursing organizations to be licensed in Georgia. It evolved from an organization founded in 1897 called the *Hospital of the Atlanta Circle of the King's Daughters and Sons*, which operated the "Hospital for Incurables," also referred to as the "Home for Incurables" for patients suffering from incurable diseases. The title reflects a highly institutional and unfortunate history of ageism and ableism, which wasn't uncommon at that time. Titles like this would certainly be shunned today, but in yesteryears, it was the norm for similar organizations.

Volunteers who operated the Hospital for Incurables approached local Atlanta businessman and philanthropist, Amos Giles Rhodes, and asked if he would donate money to replace the roof of the building. Instead, he donated both the land and funds for an entirely new building, which opened in 1904 and became the first of three A.G. Rhodes locations. That location went through a major remodel and renovation in the late 1970s, and with the exception of an added therapy gym, a renovated community room and some cosmetic improvements, it looks much the same. Two more A.G. Rhodes locations, A.G. Rhodes Cobb and A.G. Rhodes Wesley Woods, were built in the 1990s, and all three of our locations still bear resemblance to hospitals. This is typical for most of our nation's nursing homes and the environmental design leaves much to be desired.

Today, after decades of positive evolution, our three homes still bear relics of a highly institutional physical plant design that characterize many facets of our industry. Perhaps the best examples of this are our long hallways and nurse stations on each floor. Anywhere from forty to forty-eight residents reside on one floor, and they dine in huge dining rooms that accommodate up to one hundred residents. Among our three locations, we can accommodate up to 418 residents in our 259 rooms. Only one hundred of our rooms are private rooms, which means that most of our residents have roommates and share bathing and toileting facilities.

Despite its design challenges, A.G. Rhodes has done a tremendous job in our nearly 120-year history of being among the top nursing home organizations in Georgia. We have a history of excellent health care inspections and strong quality indicators. As one of only a few mission-driven nonprofit nursing home providers, we also boast the nonprofit difference where surplus revenue is put directly back into resident care and staff in the form of programs, improvements, and benefits. Although we still operate in a traditional nursing home setting, we are a community of choice in metro Atlanta.

A.G. Rhodes has always embraced technology and we're often early adopters. We were one of the first nursing home providers in Georgia to convert from paper to Electric Medical Record (EMR) charting years before it was popular or required. We feature innovative programming, including two signature programs: horticultural therapy and music therapy, which are the most transformative programs I've seen in my twenty-plus years in the industry.

Several years before the pandemic, we began a journey to improve our model of care by implementing a person-directed or person-centered model. As a testament to this, all three of our homes were accepted into the Eden Alternative Registry, which is a distinction for organizations showing a strong commitment to transforming traditional approaches to care through a person-directed approach. Prior to COVID-19, our homes thrived in their respective markets and maintained occupancy levels of nearly 95 percent.

For all our hard work and fine reputation, even A.G. Rhodes lacks consumer appeal for today's elders and for the son or daughter who is likely making the decision on where to place their loved one. The sad reality is that unlike buying a home or choosing an assisted living community, the decision to move into a nursing home is usually made quickly under extreme duress.

Nursing home complexities

In most cases, an elder will come to a nursing home after having an acute illness or accident requiring hospitalization. With declining reimbursements and disincentives for hospitals keeping patients too long, an elder's family is forced to make a quick decision on where their loved one needs to go after their hospital stay. Consumers are given a list of three to four nursing homes to choose from, sometimes less, and the consumer may be deliberately steered in the direction of one home because of established relationships with the hospital or its discharge planning staff.

Some homes are in higher demand than others which may result in no availability, and consumers are also challenged to find care that is covered by whatever complicated insurance plan they have. Most residents don't have an insurance plan or the financial means to cover more than a short-term stay in a nursing home, and if long-term care is required, they must look to Medicaid for coverage.

Nursing homes today also care for much sicker residents than in years past and the average resident has multiple comorbidities and underlying chronic conditions. Given that they demand greater clinical oversight, it's no wonder most nursing homes look and feel more like hospitals.

These factors are further complicated by the extreme regulatory burdens placed on nursing homes, and our industry ranks as one of the highest regulated by governmental oversight. Many put it as the third highest regulated after the nuclear and airline industries. There are numerous regulatory threads that run through the operations and governance of nursing homes. We are regulated by a web of local, state, and federal entities that sometimes have inconsistent requirements which makes nursing home management challenging.

The flowchart below was prepared by Jason Bring, health care law partner at Arnold Golden Gregory. I find it useful to show the many agencies with oversight of nursing homes. Because many of these agencies do not report to or work regularly with one another, the burden is on nursing home providers to navigate a complicated bureaucratic workflow.

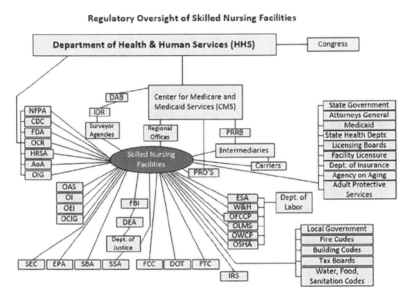

Regulatory Oversight of Skilled Nursing Facilities

My observations should not imply that we do away with nursing home regulatory agencies or regulations. Regulations are extremely important in creating a much-needed framework for operations and establishing standards for safety and quality of care that reflect the most current research and science. The importance of regulations designed to ensure and protect the rights of our residents and staff cannot be understated and need to carry with them a strong arm of enforcement to ensure compliance. However, there is an alarming frequency to which new regulations are thrust on providers, which comes at a significant financial and operational cost.

Several years ago, our federal regulatory agency, the Centers for Medicare and Medicaid Services (CMS), announced new regulations for nursing homes in the form of new phases of Requirements of Participation (ROPs) as well as a complete overhaul to our payment system. Many of the ROPs involved extreme and unrealistic documentation requirements and carried a high price tag to an industry that already operates with low margins. CMS estimated that these unfunded mandates would cost $831 million the first year with an ongoing annual cost of $736 million. In Georgia, this came out to an estimated cost of $22 million the first year and $19 million each year after.

What was more concerning for us was that the new documentation requirements would divert time and attention away from resident care. The focus was on paper compliance rather than bedside care. As A.G. Rhodes was moving toward person-directed care, we needed to focus care, resources, and attention closest to the resident and not on administrative and office duties.

Regulatory burdens create even more tension in an already high-stress, complicated industry, and they impede real improvements in our industry. The demands that regulations have placed on providers has made change and innovation a very difficult proposition for many. In such a fast-paced regulatory environment, federal and state regulations have in some cases stifled visionary and strategic thinking.

An overabundance of regulations also leaves too many opportunities for them to be improperly prioritized and inconsistently enforced. Many regulations simply do not achieve their intended purposes of safeguarding residents and staff, and in fact, they negatively impact their well-being. Providers end up becoming too rigid and inflexible in their care and protection of our nation's seniors. More regulations do not necessarily correlate with safer nursing homes. Further, the concept of "surplus of safety" has haunted us for decades and has severely inhibited innovation and creative enterprise in our industry.

In December 2017, A.G. Rhodes was asked to host Seema Verma, the former Administrator of CMS, who was in town to meet with providers and affirm the administration's goals to reduce unnecessary regulatory burdens or "putting paperwork over patients." I was asked to moderate a panel of nursing home administrators, physicians, and direct care staff. We were all encouraged by Administrator Verma's visit and conceptually we all agreed that some regulatory reduction was needed. Although a well-intentioned visit, providers have seen very little relief and we've simply learned to live with these encumbrances.

Like many other industries in this country, ours is also highly litigious. Nursing home lawsuits have been on the rise for years. You can simply open a newspaper or turn on the television to see an abundance of paid advertising aimed at consumers who have loved ones in nursing homes. The nursing home insurance market has responded with draconian premium and deductible increases, stricter underwriting standards, and a general reluctance to cover many organizations because of the innate risk profile of the industry.

COVID-19 has inflated these liability issues. Although many states, including Georgia, have passed liability protection, the liability we may face when the crisis subsides is top of mind for the industry and its insurers. Just a few of many liability considerations include how quickly a facility locked down to outside visitors, how strictly the facilities followed proper policies and procedures to contain the virus' spread, if exposed and asymptomatic workers spread the virus unknowingly, challenges controlling the spread of the virus, lack of treatment options for patients, staffing shortages because of infection, refusal to come to work or walkouts, and lack of adequate Personal Protective Equipment (PPE) (https://www.insurancejournal.com/news/national/2020/05/10/567421.htm).

Whether or not there is a correlation between lawsuits and quality of care is debatable, but what is certain is that nursing homes are easy targets for legal claims and this trend shows no signs of improvement. Sadly, the forecast among insurance companies and plaintiffs' attorneys are that claims related to COVID-19 are going to significantly impact the liability market for years to come. Difficult judicial jurisdictions like Georgia—which the American Tort Reform (ATF) foundation recently named as a top ten "Judicial Hellhole" for 2020–2021—will likely see early signs of this as insurance renewals come around during the pandemic period (http://www.judicialhellholes.org/reports/).

Perfect COVID conditions

As we reflect on COVID-19's devastating and sudden impact on our nursing homes, we must consider the historical, societal, and industry complexities that intensified this crisis. Unfortunately, the residents living in our nation's nursing homes have been most unfairly impacted by our outdated physical plants and ever-increasing regulatory and litigious burdens. All these realities became fodder for the spread of COVID-19, even for the highest-quality providers.

On that February morning when I learned that some of our nation's first to be impacted by COVID-19 were nursing home residents and staff, I knew that we were in for a true challenge. Nursing homes were easily the "ground zero" of all fifty states. Some states, when faced with the challenge of a deficit in hospital beds because of rising cases, insisted on nursing homes being more open to accepting patients with COVID-19 from the hospitals. Some even operationalized this with strict policies and guidelines. Understandably, this would relieve the growing strain on hospital bed availability, but it essentially moved the frying pan to the fire.

All the conditions were just right—enough fuel, oxygen, and combustible material was present for this brushfire to start, spread, and ravage us for over a year. It didn't take a psychic to see what was about to happen. The script was written years before the play was cast.

Chapter 2

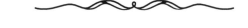

A Tale of Three Nursing Homes

According to the American Health Care Association, 70 percent of the nation's nursing homes are operated by for-profit companies compared to 24 percent by nonprofits and 6 percent operated by government agencies. A.G. Rhodes is one of the few nonprofit nursing home providers in Georgia. Each of our homes has a designated 501c3 nonprofit status, and the organization is centrally managed by A.G. Rhodes Management, which has its own 501c3 status. We are governed by a two-tiered board system with a board of trustees and a board of advisors that promote, support, and further our charitable mission.

As a testament to our mission-driven, nonprofit status, all three of our homes are dually certified to provide services to Medicare and Medicaid beneficiaries. Regardless of socioeconomic status, we are guided by what is best for the physical, social, and psychological well-being of our patients and residents.

While all three of our homes are in metro Atlanta, each operates in a different county which differs culturally, demographically, and economically. Because our homes are unique to the communities in which they reside, this can create centralized management challenges as operations can't always be executed in a one-size-fits-all approach. Despite our unique differences, we consider ourselves "One A.G. Rhodes" to realize our mission of providing expert and compassionate rehabilitation therapy and residential care to seniors in metro Atlanta.

A.G. Rhodes Atlanta

The first of our homes opened in 1904 near the Grant Park neighborhood of Atlanta in Fulton County. Today, our legacy home, with a 138-bed capacity, still stands on the corner of Woodward Avenue and Boulevard. A.G. Rhodes Atlanta proudly reflects the mission of the organization in its purest form with nearly 85 percent of the resident population receiving Medicaid.

A.G. Rhodes Atlanta serves a more than 90 percent Black resident population and more than 90 percent of its staff are Black. Although this location has the most physical plant challenges because of its age, ironically it has the most private room accommodations with forty-four private rooms. Because of this, A.G. Rhodes Atlanta avoided significant COVID-19 infection for nine months before they too experienced outbreaks in December 2020.

Of our three locations, the Atlanta home serves the fewest number of patients needing subacute rehabilitation services despite its capacity to do so in its state-of-the-art rehab gym built in 2011. This gym features one of the only aquatic therapy pools in a nursing home in Georgia, which provides a significant community service to those needing aquatic therapy exercise and treatments.

Admittedly, this home is my sentimental favorite not only because of its unique history, but because I was the administrator there for eight years.

A.G. Rhodes Cobb

Based on the incredible success of our Atlanta home, it was only natural that the organization would seek to extend its reach and services to meet increasing needs in the community. In the early 1990s, we received a Certificate of Need (CON) to build a 130-bed facility in Marietta, a large city and suburb just outside of Atlanta located in Cobb County, Georgia. This location opened in 1992.

Although built in the early nineties, A.G. Rhodes Cobb was still built on a traditional nursing home model. This location has only eighteen private rooms among two floors with long hallways and large nursing stations. A.G. Rhodes Cobb has communal dining, communal shower rooms, and most of the other medical model design elements that characterize nursing homes.

Similar to the demographic makeup of the county, the Cobb facility serves a majority White resident population, nearly 80 percent. Most of its staff are Black and other minorities. About 60 percent of the A.G. Rhodes Cobb residents receive Medicaid.

A.G. Rhodes Cobb was the first of our communities to be accepted to the Eden Alternative Registry and they boast a culture where person-directed practices seem organic. Despite an increasingly difficult regulatory environment, the Cobb home has accomplished successful state and federal regulatory surveys year over year. Cobb also enjoys an affiliation agreement with Wellstar Hospital— the largest hospital system in the county—which provides medical direction and other clinical services to the facility.

A.G. Rhodes Wesley Woods

A.G. Rhodes Wesley Woods—a 150-bed facility—opened in 1997 near Atlanta's Emory University Hospital in DeKalb County. This location is nestled on Emory's Wesley Woods campus and was built through a lease agreement with Emory. The building sits on leased land and provides much-needed skilled nursing care to the community and pays Emory for medical direction, clinical services, and pastoral services.

It's obvious that A.G. Rhodes Wesley Woods operates on a medical campus. It's commonplace to see hospital physicians in training and medical specialists all donning lab coats. Because of its relationship with the hospital, A.G. Rhodes Wesley Woods sees constant admissions and discharges and its business model relies heavily on patients who need short-term, subacute rehabilitation services.

Wesley Woods serves a 60 percent White resident population and a nearly 40 percent Black resident population. Approximately

90 percent of the staff are Black, and approximately 10 percent are White. Wesley Woods has thirty-eight private rooms and is the only one of our communities with a dedicated unit that cares for people living with dementia. The building has four floors and like our other homes, it has the traditional nursing home characteristics.

A.G. Rhodes Management

The A.G. Rhodes Management Company was formed in 2012. For the previous thirty years, A.G. Rhodes was managed by a contract management company, Bauguess Management, founded by Harve Bauguess. Harve is a pioneering figure in Georgia's nursing home industry and was instrumental in A.G. Rhodes' expansion and impact in metro Atlanta. When Harve retired, the board of trustees voted to form an in-house management company to oversee the management responsibilities of the organization.

When A.G. Rhodes Management's first CEO was hired, Al Blackwelder, he brought on the organization's first fundraising/development director and communications officer—two vital roles for any thriving nonprofit. For the next several years, the management office would undergo changes to centralize and streamline several areas of our operations more effectively. In 2019, the management office changed its name to the support office to reflect that its primary purpose is to support the operations in the homes.

Program expansion: music therapy and horticultural therapy

In 2014, Emory Healthcare closed the rehabilitation services at their Wesley Woods Hospital, which is located on the same campus as our A.G. Rhodes Wesley Woods nursing home. Al was CEO at the time, and he seized this fruitful opportunity to hire two therapists there whose programs would no longer be offered: a horticultural therapist and a music therapist. A.G. Rhodes would now be among very few homes to offer these innovative programs in skilled nursing. Additionally, since the Wesley Woods Hospital would no longer have horticultural therapy, two greenhouses were transferred from Emory to our Atlanta and Cobb communities.

Music therapy incorporates musical activities to address physical, emotional, cognitive, and social needs of individuals. Activities such as singing, moving, or listening to music can help improve speech, motor skills, memory, and balance. Our director of music therapy and certified music therapist, John Abel, spends time at each home administering music therapy in group and individual settings. Treatment may take place at bedside, in resident living areas, and in general activity spaces.

With the vast musical experience and interest of our patients and residents, John incorporates music from the 1920s to the present day. Styles range from big band jazz, country, religious, rock 'n' roll, and old-time sing-alongs. The way in which patients engage in music depends on their level of functioning and treatment goals. Several common music therapy practices involve singing, moving to music, playing instruments, or listening.

In addition to the clinical benefits, music therapy sessions are fun, motivating, and lighthearted while encompassing the personal musical preferences of the patients. Co-treatment between music therapy and other therapies including physical, occupational, and speech occurs on a weekly basis. In addition to interfacing with other rehabilitation therapies, John works in conjunction with staff from the activities, restorative, and nursing departments. Patient goals may vary from improved speech (through singing), balance, or strength to increased motivation or attention.

Our director of horticultural therapy and registered horticultural therapist, Kirk Hines, incorporates horticultural activities designed to achieve specific and documented treatment goals. For example, planting herbs helps increase sensory stimulation, watering helps improve motor skills, and group gardening helps decrease isolation and depression. Like John, Kirk travels to each of our homes throughout the week to work with groups and individuals, and sessions take place in resident living areas, in general activity spaces, in the therapeutic gardens, greenhouses, or at bedside. Patients engage in planting, sowing seeds, taking cuttings, and light garden maintenance during their sessions. The program's physical structures include therapeutic gardens, greenhouses, and indoor fluorescent light units. There are planters of varying heights, fragrant plants, paved surfaces, water features, and meditation space located in the gardens. The climate-controlled greenhouses are designed for walker and wheelchair mobility, and sitting and standing-height benches help facilitate gardening to accommodate patients at various functional levels. Surrounding the greenhouses are therapeutic gardens with heirloom plants that stimulate the senses and help recall past memories. Visitors and family members are also encouraged to visit the greenhouse and gardens for a relaxing change of scenery and relief from stress. In the group rooms and rehabilitation therapy gym, portable fluorescent light carts are used for indoor gardening which enable residents and patients to nurture their new cuttings and seedlings regardless of the weather outside.

Upon discharge, patients take home their seedlings, cuttings, and transplants in order to continue the leisure interest that began or was reintroduced during rehabilitation at A.G. Rhodes. Co-treatment between horticultural therapy and other therapies including physical, occupational, and speech occurs on a weekly basis. During treatment, patient needs are assessed and goals are established. Horticultural therapy may assist by increasing activity level, reintegration into a past interest, or by decreasing stress and anxiety.

These therapies are components of our therapy and rehabilitation department; however, they are not reimbursed through Medicare, Medicaid, or insurance. Regardless, they have undeniable qualitative and quantitative outcomes and have become staple programs for our residents. To ensure these important programs continue, we enlist the community to help us raise funds through "Songs for Seniors" and "Seeds for Seniors" fundraising campaigns. In 2018, a new greenhouse was built at A.G. Rhodes Wesley Woods, thanks in large part to these philanthropic efforts.

Our journey to person-directed care

Several years ago, we began researching different models of care nationally and internationally that better align quality care and quality of life as inseparable and equally important factors in all aspects of a resident's daily living. Our goal was to explore best practices that we might implement at A.G. Rhodes.

An A.G. Rhodes team traveled to the Netherlands and visited several communities that embraced the household model, which is a smaller model of care where fewer residents live in a community that they recognize as home. In the models we toured, we observed varying numbers of residents per household with different staffing patterns, including models that had employees working in traditional departments and those that had universal workers. In each example, the feeling of family and community was clear, and we knew instantly that this was what we wanted to see at A.G. Rhodes.

Another notable observation from the Netherlands was how much respect and reverence existed for older adults. I am often asked about my biggest takeaway from our visit to the Netherlands and my answer is always the same: they have a sophisticated culture and value system regarding elders. Nursing home residents, and elders in general, are viewed as an integral part of the community. Additionally, their approach to volunteerism is something I have never seen before. Volunteering is a part of the Dutch fabric, and it is well documented that a significant segment of the population is involved in volunteer activities. The nursing homes we visited were buzzing with activity and one could not differentiate between a volunteer or a staff member. Additionally, many nurses in training volunteer at nursing homes which undoubtedly assists the labor force and increases the sense of community.

One nursing home we visited had only a short row of shrubbery separating the nursing home from the general community. We were surprised by this because we could easily see how a resident could wander away. I asked the director if residents ever wandered away, and he replied that they occasionally do but that neighbors always bring them back. I am not making a case for nursing homes in the US to assume the same protocols, but it was heartwarming to see how the community in general revered older adults.

Upon returning to the US, we did a similar exploratory process and toured many of our nation's household models. The Leonard

Florence Center for living in Chelsea, Massachusetts, was one that stood out. It's a Green House community—a small home model nursing home with all private rooms—which was of particular interest to us because it was the first urban Green House. Ironically, the day we visited that community, it was having its annual state and federal survey inspection. We were impressed with the staff's business-as-usual attitude during the survey, which is normally a stressful process for nursing home staff. Our tour and meetings continued while the surveyors conducted their inspection. This was the type of management culture regarding regulators that we aspired to. It should be noted that their inspection resulted in a deficiency-free survey.

After touring communities and gathering best practices, in 2016 we decided to embark on our journey into practicing person-directed care, which frames and prioritizes the delivery of care according to the needs and preferences of our residents versus prioritizing operational or staff efficiencies. We enlisted the support of the Eden Alternative® to guide us, and by 2018, all three homes were accepted into the Eden Alternative Registry.

We continue to strive for continuous quality improvement through person-directed care. We take a collaborative approach to care which hinges on the belief that all members of a care partnership team are equally involved and important in the planning and delivery of care. This care partnership draws on the resources and skills from staff, other health care professionals, families, friends, volunteers, others in the community, and most importantly, the elders themselves. The relationships fostered are mutually beneficial and meaningful to all and we work together to achieve higher-quality care and a more meaningful quality of life.

While we are still early in our efforts to completely transform to a person-directed model of care, we are determined to create environments of care which are not only biomedical but consider all aspects of a resident's wellbeing.

Care partnership philosophy depiction

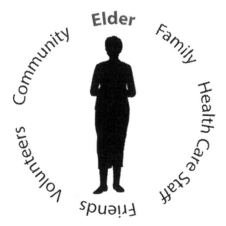

A.G. Rhodes timeline

- 1897: The Hospital of the Atlanta Circle of the King's Daughters and Sons is founded on Church Street, Now Carnegie Way.
- 1900: Hospital officials ask Amos Giles Rhodes, founder of Rhodes Furniture, for funding to make repairs. Instead, Mr. Rhodes provides land and funding needed for a new building.
- 1904: Construction is complete, and the hospital reopens at the corner of Boulevard and Woodward Avenues, where today's flagship home is located.
- 1930: In conjunction with a major renovation, the home was renamed after Mr. Rhodes who passed away two years prior.
- 1992: A.G. Rhodes opens its Cobb home.
- 1997: A.G. Rhodes opens its Wesley Woods Home.
- 2010: A.G. Rhodes Atlanta completes a significant renovation resulting in the addition of a therapy and rehabilitation gym.

- 2011: A.G. Rhodes continues to expand subacute and rehabilitation services at Cobb and Wesley Woods locations.
- 2014: A.G. Rhodes adds music therapy and horticultural therapy to its programming.
- 2016: A.G. Rhodes enters a partnership with the Eden Alternative® to train and educate staff in person-directed care, particularly for people living with dementia.
- 2018: All three homes are accepted into the Eden Alternative Registry, making A.G. Rhodes the first standalone nursing home organization in Georgia with this status.
- 2019: The A.G. Rhodes management office becomes the A.G. Rhodes Support Office.
- 2021: A.G. Rhodes embarks on a capital campaign to raise funds for environmental improvements at our Cobb home.

Chapter 3

April Fools

On April 1, 2020, the first COVID-19 case emerged at A.G. Rhodes. By this time, COVID-19 already began ravaging nursing homes in metro Atlanta, so we knew it was not a matter of if but when. With our limited testing supplies, we started testing symptomatic residents and clenched our teeth as we desperately hoped and prayed the tests would be negative. When I received a call that our Wesley Woods home had its first case, my heart sank. Resident cases there quickly rose to seven within the first week.

By that time, strict visitation limitations had been in place and were required for all nursing homes since mid-March 2020. Visitation would only be allowed in compassionate care situations which were somewhat loosely defined by CMS as follows:

> For ALL *facilities nationwide: Facilities should restrict visitation of all visitors and non-essential health care personnel, except for certain compassionate care situations, such as an end-of-life situation. In those cases, visitors will be limited to a specific room only. Facilities are expected to notify potential visitors to defer visitation until further notice (through signage, calls, letters, etc.). Note: If a state implements actions that exceed CMS requirements, such as a ban on all visitation through a governor's*

executive order, a facility would not be out of compliance with CMS' requirements. In this case, surveyors would still enter the facility but not cite for noncompliance with visitation requirements.

For individuals that enter in compassionate situations (e.g., end-of-life care), facilities should require visitors to perform hand hygiene and use Personal Protective Equipment (PPE), such as facemasks. Decisions about visitation during an end-of-life situation should be made on a case-by-case basis, which should include careful screening of the visitor (including clergy, bereavement counselors, etc.) for fever or respiratory symptoms. Those with symptoms of a respiratory infection (fever, cough, shortness of breath, or sore throat) should not be permitted to enter the facility at any time (even in end-of-life situations). Those visitors that are permitted must wear a facemask while in the building and restrict their visit to the resident's room or other location designated by the facility. They should also be reminded to frequently perform hand hygiene. QSO-20-14-NH.

Recognizing the severe toll of isolation and separation on residents and families, CMS issued guidance in June 2020 that would allow nursing homes to accommodate very controlled indoor and outdoor visitation. Visitation would be allowed if two conditions were met: the county positivity rate (the percentage of all COVID-19 tests performed in that county which were positive) had to be below a certain percentage for at least ten days, and the nursing home had to be out of outbreak status for at least fourteen days.

A.G. Rhodes' three homes are located in highly dense counties, and throughout the pandemic, they had some of the highest positivity rates in the state. Also, because an outbreak is defined as one more positive case, our homes could accommodate very limited visitation opportunities throughout the height of the pandemic.

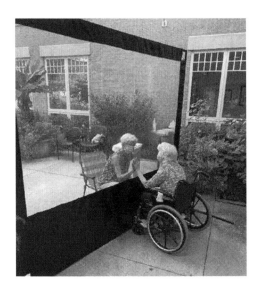

I still recall our first outdoor visit at our Wesley Woods home in August after four months of being closed to families and visitors. The visitation area was set up on a patio space outside the facility with a tall, clear screen we purchased to separate visitors from residents for their health and safety. The daughter of one of our residents arrived with her folding chair, which we asked visitors to bring as a precaution to limit possible spread of infection. After completing the required COVID-19 screening, she sat on one side of the screen. A staff member brought her mother to the other side of the screen where she sat in her wheelchair. Both wearing masks, the two tearfully stretched their arms and each brought the palms of their hands up to touch the other's with the screen in between. A staff member took a picture of the touching moment, and it has become emblematic of the pain and separation caused by COVID-19 and the sad reality that our nation's nursing home residents and families experienced for many months.

COVID-19 preparations:

Nursing home staff have long been trained on disaster management and emergency procedures, especially following Hurricane

Katrina in 2005. After more recent crises, training requirements have increased in most states. Disaster training is usually in the form of tabletop exercises, and as a team, we draw on best practices to work through various disaster scenarios. For example, a natural disaster that causes damage and brings the power down or an evacuation following a simulated chemical spill from a train that ran off the track and leaked toxic chemicals near the nursing home. No amount of disaster training could have adequately prepared us for this pandemic. Nursing home staff also go through extensive and continuous training in infection control and standard precautions. We are also accustomed to isolation procedures and vaccine distribution related to long and difficult flu seasons. Again, our vast experience in these areas were not enough to properly equip us against the extraordinary challenges of COVID-19.

When the World Health Organization defined COVID-19 as a pandemic, we first saw the impact through our supply chain. Almost overnight, we could no longer get basic supplies and PPE such as masks, gloves, and gowns. Because these items were normally so easy to obtain and some were not as routinely used in our settings, we seldom kept large quantities on hand. The recommended face mask protection for COVID-19 was an N95 particulate respirator mask. These masks were designed to fit very closely to the face and form a seal, protecting the nose and mouth. The N95 was particularly effective at filtering airborne particles, thus preventing the spread of infection. Prior to COVID-19, these masks would cost between eighty cents and $1, depending on the quantity ordered, but the cost skyrocketed to $5 in a matter of days and largely were not available from traditional suppliers.

In mid-April, one of our administrators told me about a training on COVID-19 precautions that he arranged at his facility. On showing me the slide deck for the training, I noticed it contained the proper method to "fit test" an N95 prior to wearing. This prompted me to ask for an inventory of how many of these masks we had as an organization. The results of the inventory were shocking. We only had a few N95 masks on hand per home and our suppliers were all reporting that because of the crisis, all of their masks in stock were federally quarantined. Similarly, we couldn't find disposable gowns, gloves, face shields, or hand sanitizer. You name it, and we probably couldn't get it.

The situation with masks was so critical that early on in the crisis, the Centers for Disease Control and Prevention (CDC) issued recommendations for reusing masks. Masks were not manufactured for reuse, but because of the shortages, providers had no choice. Early on in the crisis, the CDC also approved the use of KN95 masks as an alternative. KN95 masks were considered the Chinese alternative to N95 masks, but there was less data available about their testing standards or filtration efficacy. Later, the federal government would contract with organizations to clean and decontaminate used masks. We were, as the saying goes, "deep in it."

Unscrupulous individuals began profiting off our misfortune by hoarding supplies to sell on the "black market." When we tried to get supplies from local retail stores like Home Depot, Lowe's, or Grainger, nothing was on the shelves. When you could find items, quantities were extremely low and the stores imposed limits. Some stores had inventory at other locations or in their warehouses, but whenever we tried to place an order, supplies were blocked and designated as quarantined pandemic supply. Even when showing identification and work credentials, many would refuse to sell us large quantities.

We were forced to purchase whatever small quantities we could, and we went to several stores each day to buy whatever was available. We had to improvise, using whatever we could to get the job done. We used painter suits as gowns, swim goggles as eye protection, and gaiters as masks. We became adept at making do with what we had.

Drinking from the fire hose

By the end of April, we had forty cumulative resident cases and twenty-eight cumulative staff cases among our three buildings. Sadly, six residents died. Miraculously, our flagship location near Grant Park—which serves a more than 90 percent Black resident population, the most at-risk population—had no resident cases.

Our support team held daily calls with the homes, and we were doing whatever we could to contain the virus. No idea was a bad one; we were open to suggestions. Best practices from one home were replicated in another, and failed ideas were discarded. The situation was evolving so quickly, and significant time was devoted to communicating with residents, their families, and staff. We tried to update them each step of the way. We were following ever-changing guidance from several federal and state agencies, and it was difficult to keep up. The information was coming at us through a fire hose. We would often hear about new CDC recommendations on the news at night and we could only brace ourselves because invariably these recommendations would become guidance or policy by the following day. It was difficult to stay ahead, but we kept trying.

As staff cases began to rise, staffing of our homes became a serious concern. We have always prided ourselves in avoiding using outside agency staffing. Based on our person-directed philosophy, agency staff do not provide sufficient consistency to truly get to know our residents or individualize care. Another big issue was that the cost of using a staff agency resulted in three to four times what we pay our regular staff. Not only was this an obvious financial concern, but it presented serious implications to staff morale. However, out of sheer necessity, we scrambled to sign agency contracts to ensure that if we got to a critical staffing point, we would have a plan to fall back on. Fortuitously but more importantly, thanks to our strong culture, we did not have to rely on many agency staff.

Because of our physical layout and our deficit in private rooms, an early logistical issue became our ability to isolate residents who were being treated or monitored for COVID-19. Even if residents in isolation tested negative for the virus, we had to assume they were exposed and potentially positive because of the intubation period associated with the virus. We could relax isolation procedures only when we could confirm that they weren't contagious. This was the only way to slow the spread of the virus. Like most in the industry, we constructed temporary units to aide isolation. These isolation units were quickly constructed and were rudimentary. We had several types of units, each serving different purposes at different times:

one for those with active COVID-19 infection (COVID units) and others to house residents who were under observation, such as residents who were newly admitted to A.G. Rhodes who could have been exposed at the hospital or elsewhere prior to admission.

Our Cobb community had constructed one such unit only to have an officer with the local fire department—which is one of the many entities that enforces regulations in nursing homes—come that same night and tell them to remove it immediately. He deemed it a fire hazard. I called the officer myself to explain that we had to isolate residents to save lives. I asked him for an alternative and his response was that we had to draw up plans and submit them to his office for approval. I could not believe what I was hearing. We were "damned if we do, damned if we don't." We took down the walls and turned the entire floor into an isolation unit.

These units had significant consequences. They forced us to turn semi-private rooms into private rooms thus severely impacting our occupancy. Our occupancy levels fell to below 70 percent. This seriously impacted revenue and threatened our survival. More importantly, it displaced many residents from their rooms which had profound effects especially for those living with dementia. We were forced to abruptly relocate residents from their familiar surroundings, in many cases, to a new floor where different staff would be caring for them.

When will this end?

When was this going to end? That was the question we asked ourselves every day. Many assumed the virus would die off as the weather warmed up as experience has shown other viruses don't withstand the heat. Reports of lab experiments suggested that heat and humidity killed the virus. But prevailing opinions on the news was that COVID-19 would continue to rise if the general public didn't follow sound standard precautions like wearing masks, social distancing, and washing and sanitizing hands. Initially, masks were thought to prevent the wearer from spreading the virus, but it was later proven to prevent both the spread and contracting of COVID-19. While nursing home staff were required to wear masks, mask wearing and social distancing weren't universally accepted or adopted by others.

As each month went by, we thought we were inching closer to the pandemic's end. We would closely follow any ebbs or flows of community infection rates. We each had our own theories on when and how it would subside, but none of us would have imagined that it would continue into a new year and have some of its highest infection rates in early 2021. In February 2021, the Atlanta Journal Constitution published the article, "In Spite of Months in COVID Lockdown, GA Senior Care Homes Report Highest Deaths, Cases in January" (https://www.ajc.com/news/coronavirus/in-spite-of-months-in-covid-lockdown-senior-care-homes-report-highest-deaths-cases-in-january).

The public scrutiny, which was squarely on us when the pandemic began, continued almost a year later. Due to COVID-19 surges in the community, in January 2021, long-term care communities in Georgia reported the highest one-month total for positive cases and deaths since the start of the pandemic. This was after having almost no visitation for most of those months. The media reported continued issues with public reporting of COVID-19 cases and deaths. New York, which arguably had the most notoriety for its handling of the COVID-19 virus and its openness and transparency in reporting, was later slammed in the national press and political and public quarters for allegedly withholding data regarding thousands of deaths. Ironically, New York was one of the states that strongly and publicly insisted on the transfer of infected and contagious hospital patients to nursing homes to relieve the pressure and increase the supply of hospital beds.

The public specter of COVID-19 on our nation's nursing homes and their COVID-19 response was not going away nor was the increased policy and regulatory burdens that would result. Now, policies related to testing, isolation, cohorting, cleaning, and disinfecting are likely to become permanently ingrained into the fabric of nursing home operations.

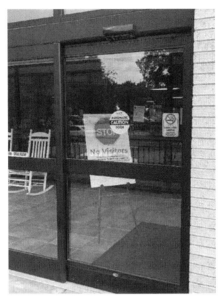

Entrances to our buildings were closed to visitors.

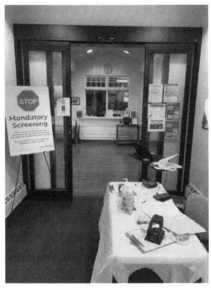

*Staff and essential personnel must complete screening
process at stations set up at each location.*

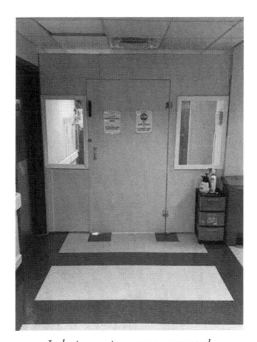

Isolation units were constructed.

Chapter 4

Leadership in Times of Crisis

Leadership matters and it matters most at difficult times.
—Former 1st Lt. John Frazer, US Army

To call this a book about leadership would be grossly misrepresenting its content, however, I want to highlight a few of the leadership lessons I learned during this crisis.

The quote above is from John Frazer, a member of the A.G. Rhodes board of trustees and its executive committee. John is a former army ranger, and since his time in the military, he's had an impressive banking career. He led SunTrust (now Truist) bank operations in Memphis and now he's a highly successful wealth and investment advisor in Atlanta.

When John would utter these words to me long before COVID-19, I saw them as a gesture of appreciation, inspiration, support, and guidance. Sometimes, he would close an e-mail with those words, and sometimes over lunch, he would inject them into our conversation. I never quite processed them, but they stayed in my mental reservoir. Once the pandemic hit, these words became top of mind.

At a virtual CEO Leadership Summit in August 2020, hosted by the Chief Executive Group, Retired Marine Corps General James Mattis said, "Crises are harsh auditors of character." COVID-19 has exposed many leadership issues throughout businesses, organizations, cities, states, and nations. The crucial role of leadership has been on center stage more than ever before. The integrity of leaders everywhere continues to be closely scrutinized, criticized, and in many cases, publicized. COVID-19 has heightened expectations of effective leadership. Nursing home leaders are no different. As soon as COVID-19 emerged in the Washington State nursing home, we immediately knew that we would be in the spotlight and that our actions, or inactions, would be closely critiqued.

The stakes are high at nursing homes. In addition to the lives of residents and staff, the leaders of the A.G. Rhodes homes are each responsible for a $15 million book of business. Fortunately, our administrators—Kristie Davis, Melanie Haders, and Greg Heath—together have more than fifty years of nursing home experience. They were our highest-ranking officers in the field and their strong leadership was critical as they led their forces fearlessly into battle.

In early March 2020, I directed members of our support team, including our administrators and other nursing home leadership, to start having daily calls to ensure we were all operating from the same page. These morning calls helped us make consistent decisions as a team and stay current on the many regulatory guidelines and executive orders that were coming at us and changing almost daily. The calls would start with our administrators reporting the number of resident and staff cases in each home and the numbers of residents on isolation and observation. We discussed any regulatory or guidance changes, newly signed executive orders, visitation status in the homes, testing frequency and dates, communications needs or issues, supply needs or issues, and very importantly, staffing needs. After we felt more comfortable with what and when to report, we moved from daily calls to three times weekly on Mondays, Wednesdays, and Fridays.

My chief operating officer, Keith Wilson, led these calls, but I also attended as I felt it was important that I got firsthand information as it evolved. It may seem like micromanagement, but it was clear to me that in this crisis situation, I needed to know the details as soon as they were available.

We received regular press inquiries, and a few reporters knew my number and would call me directly. I also had regular conversations with my board leadership. With the situation moving so rapidly, I wanted the most current information at my fingertips. At this time, I also developed a hunger for reading, researching, and educating myself as much as I could about COVID-19 and recommended courses of action. From transmission, testing, vaccine development, isolation procedures, and more, I wanted to know it and articulate it with confidence to any given audience. Only in college had I studied this much and now I was doing it from an entirely different position of maturity and knowledge.

I was not naïve, but I was willing to question the experts until it made sense to me. I realized that my constant quest for knowledge may aggravate some who reported to me, but I was certain it was necessary. The best example of this would be cases of COVID-19. These numbers grew so rapidly, and it was difficult to track and stay updated on the details of the cases, but I needed to know. If I got a call from the media or a question from a board member, I wanted to have as close to accurate information as possible. Truth, transparency, and trust guided me each step of the way.

Transformative leadership

In my opinion, rigid leadership styles can be ineffective in a crisis situation. You can neither be too democratic, too autocratic, nor too laissez-faire. A blended leadership approach is particularly useful at these fast-paced and highly critical situations. Being nimble and thinking on the spot was important. We also didn't have time for indecision. I needed my team to understand that these times called for careful but decisive actions, and decisions must be made quickly.

I became a fan of the transformative leadership style, and I was making conscious efforts to mold my leadership in that direction. The transformational leadership style focuses on clear communication, goal setting, and employee motivation. A transformational leader is driven by a commitment to organizational objectives. Transformational leadership is inspirational, and it instills trust and confidence from staff and followers. Individuals become willing participants and are not following solely because of pay or incentive.

They are working toward a common goal or cause that is much bigger than themselves.

In transformational leadership, staff are empowered and motivated. Transformational leaders look at the big picture to truly understand the magnitude of the crisis. They approach crises situations from all angles and thus they can see pros and cons from a larger perspective. They are nimble and agile enough to manage the complexities of issues which are emerging at a break-neck speed, but they always seek advice of those closest to the situation and use a team approach before executing a response. This doesn't mean they let the team decide the response, but their counsel with the team, along with their own knowledge and experience, help inform a flexible and adaptive plan.

In a crisis like COVID-19, there was rarely a time to over litigate or pontificate a situation. Ironically, military leaders are well-known for their transformative leadership styles, which is why I include military quotes in this chapter. They resonate with our experiences at A.G. Rhodes.

The team

Leading from a position of knowledge was very important for us all. Jackie Summerlin, our director of clinical services, had become quite adept at transforming everchanging guidelines and regulations into more specific organizational protocols and policies. Mary Helton, our human resources director, would operationalize the many updates that involved staff.

Our chief financial officer, Rhett Austin, and his team had their hands full with reporting requirements for our Paycheck Protection Program (PPP) loans and other stimulus moneys received. Even amidst significantly impacted occupancy levels, they also ensured timely billing to get reimbursed for our services and ensure positive cash flow. Not to mention they paid supply vendors on immediate, net zero payment terms to ensure that our already constricted supply chain kept some level of flow.

Mary Newton, our chief communications officer, was simply indispensable and frequent communications with our many stakeholders was an extremely important aspect of our efforts. Because we're a nonprofit organization, our chief development officer, Jane Simpson, worked behind the scenes to help us most effectively use fundraising to support our efforts.

Our IT team, Justin Lenning and Andrew Sagun, were key in helping us quickly adapt to the reality that we must rely on technology since face-to-face contact simply wasn't possible. Our compliance officer, Tammy Luther, managed the many compliance, legal, and risk management implications of COVID. Her documentation responsibilities and role in ensuring we were complying with regulations in such a fast-paced environment was tantamount to any other function.

In addition to their assistance related to COVID-19, these individuals still had non-COVID-19-related jobs to perform and had to continue the functions of their positions. Financial audits needed to be completed, insurance renewals were due, an annual report needed to be produced, and Minimum Data Set (MDS) submissions needed to occur monthly, and now there were more of them. Further, prior to COVID-19, we began design plans for a major project at our Cobb location in Marietta; a new building that would be based on the household model which would afford all our elders much more comfortable, private room accommodations. Even though COVID-19 was the ultimate disruptor, we knew it was critical that planning continue, and during COVID-19, we completed the design phase.

Despite a stellar team, one important piece was missing: COVID-19 is a highly infectious disease and we needed epidemiological expertise and experience. This was new to us. Our Wesley Woods community occasionally worked with an Emory epidemiologist, Dr. Scott Fridkin. While most of our work with him was through clinical research projects prior to COVID-19, he was still very generous with his services and had advised us on several occasions in the early months of COVID-19. I asked Dr. Fridkin about formally contracting with us. Although his busy schedule wouldn't allow it, he referred us to a colleague, Dr. Sujit Suchindran, who quickly became an invaluable member of our team. Dr. Suchindran worked alongside the medical directors of our three communities to ensure decisions made were based on the most current medical knowledge.

Supplies:

Because supply chains were virtually cut off at the start of this crisis, my COO, Keith, and I decided to take over the ordering of critical supplies like masks, gowns, sanitizer, face shields, cleaning supplies, and other items. These supplies were already in short demand and needed very large quantity order guarantees from suppliers. We assumed that our roles as CEO and COO would make it easier to source these since we had the budgetary authority and purchasing power to order on the spot if needed. Fortunately, we were right. Perhaps more importantly, this approach aligned with our support team philosophy. We took the time-consuming burden of ordering supplies off the administrators which allowed them to focus more attention on ensuring the safety and well-being of their residents and staff. I also had very good luck in finding some independent suppliers, individuals who could source critical supplies and PPE privately and would sell them to me directly. Some would mark them up marginally and others had mercenary profits in mind. As much as I did not want to pay the higher price tag, we needed all that we could get.

A proud moment for me was when my seventeen-year-old daughter, Kiana, volunteered to help me make face shields. We bought the supplies, and during an April weekend, she and I made more than two hundred reusable, high-quality (if I do say so myself) shields. Many others in the community exhibited similar acts of pure kindness and citizenship. A former board member, Ted Benning, owned a construction company and donated some precious N95 masks, which at that point where the hottest commodity in town. If you could get them, you would likely be paying five times regular unit price. Another current board member, Sherry Kaelin, enlisted the services of her mother, Nan Pitcher, to make cloth masks with filters as added protection.

My wife's cousin, Lorna, worked for the City of New York and put me in contact with some of her suppliers which helped us source scarce supplies. Many, many others in the community would simply drive up to the homes and donate supplies. Through *The Thanks Mom and Dad Foundation*, an Atlanta-based foundation, students from Georgia State University donated gallons and gallons of hand sanitizer. The Atlanta foundations and philanthropic community on a whole were extremely generous to us. I take every chance I can to publicly state that I would not have wanted to be in any other city than Atlanta during a crisis like this.

Supply runs gave Keith and I another great opportunity to show leadership and boost morale because we would deliver them weekly to the homes. This ensured that we were visible to our staff on the frontlines. We were truly all in this together. We were not afraid to come to the homes, and we were determined to equip staff with every supply, protection, and tool available to help them fight this enemy.

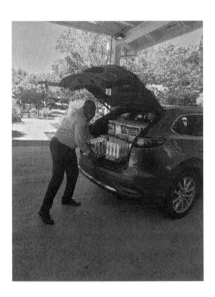

Tough leadership decision

Early in the pandemic, we faced a leadership challenge when several administrative staff asked to work from home. This practice was widely accepted and generally encouraged in most industries. We allowed some administrative staff who had preexisting conditions to do so, but now others wanted the same courtesy. We made the difficult decision to deny many of these requests. A typical nursing home usually has its administrative offices located at the building's entrance. One had to pass through those areas to get to the care units. We asked ourselves, "What impact will it have on staff morale if our direct caregivers have to walk through a virtual ghost town each day when they start their shift and put themselves in harm's way?" To make matters worse, many of the administrative staff were managers to those direct care staff.

We did work with administrative staff to offer shorter shifts and alternate days off. We followed all pertinent laws and regulations, but we wanted them present when possible. Staff understood, and ultimately, they respected our decision.

Do more with less

Indeed, COVID has disrupted routines. While our direct care staff were bravely on the frontlines, our leaders changed gears to become much more tactical and logistical. This was in response to the significantly increased infection prevention and control measures and regulatory requirements resulting from COVID. Daily screenings, weekly COVID testing for all staff and bi-weekly for residents, constant inventorying of supplies, vaccine education and distribution, and a host of other logistical needs forced us all to do more with less.

My best example of this is our volunteer and community outreach director, Kim Beasley. The volunteer program basically shut down except for a few virtual initiatives, but Kim morphed and provided direct support and assistance to our activities departments and music therapy program. Especially in a crisis, there is no room for a "That's not my job" attitude. I've been extremely impressed and proud of our team for managing this crisis with an "All hands on deck" approach.

I am a firm believer in the power of prayer, and I leaned heavily on my faith as I led through this crisis. I still pray for my leadership team each day. I pray that God will give us the wisdom, humility, understanding, and compassion to help us protect and care for our residents. I pray that we are guided by the best available science and that good judgement prevails. I pray that ambitions and egos never influence our decisions, and I pray that fear does not inhibit our prudent action. Our responsibility as leaders is critical and cannot be understated. We set the tone for the responses and the attitudes of those we lead. We must own our failures and share our successes. Ultimately, this crisis will be an arbiter of our readiness to grow as leaders in this industry.

To conclude this chapter, I reflect on a quote from Ruth Katz, senior vice president for Policy at Leading Age: "Leadership does not guarantee success, but ineffective leadership guarantees failure."

Chapter 5

Role of the Governing Body

The board—or governing body—of an organization is responsible for the organization's vison and mission. They have ultimate fiduciary responsibility and maintain oversight of the staff through the CEO. An effective board will complement an organization's leadership in areas deemed essential. Of course, they cannot and should not usurp the roles and functions of staff, but their expertise and counsel can significantly strengthen an organization.

A.G. Rhodes has a two-tiered board structure which has evolved significantly in the last two decades. The history in segregating board roles became popular in the nineteenth century but is not seen as frequently today. Even so, our boards of trustees and advisors bring significant expertise to our organization, and we benefit greatly from this two-tiered system. Many members of these boards are the second, third, and even forth generations of their family to serve, including members from prominent Atlanta families like the Perdues, Sibleys, and Parkers.

As a "green" CEO, our boards have also played an important role in my leadership development. Many members mentor me, as well as others in my leadership team, using their varied spheres of experience including governance, finance, nonprofit, human resources, management, legal, and communications to name a few. COVID-19 not only tested our staff leadership, but it challenged our boards' commitment and dedication to our mission at such a difficult time.

Both boards were up to the challenge, and this chapter details the important role they played in this crisis.

The A.G. Rhodes board of trustees is comprised of business and thought leaders in our community. The primary purpose of the trustees is to promote, support, and further the charitable mission of A.G. Rhodes. Trustees manage the affairs of the organization by overseeing business and operating plans, budgets, and capital expenditures. They support the corporation both financially and with their time. In addition, this board oversees the support office and the board of advisors.

The board of advisors serves as an advisory board to the board of trustees and makes recommendations on capital projects, community outreach, and other activities that implement and enhance the charitable purposes of A.G. Rhodes. Advisors are advocates for our organization and the issue of aging. They serve as ambassadors for our homes, supporting the organization with their time and financial contributions. They provide valuable insight to the board of trustees and maintain a strong presence in each of our homes.

The chairman of our board of trustees is David L. Perdue (no relation to the politician). David is the great-great-grandson of our company's benefactor and namesake, Amos Giles Rhodes. David is the quintessential Southern gentleman with the charm, personality, and confidence to fill any room he walks into. Extremely eloquent and always the optimist, David naturally inspires most of my team to duty. One of his favorite calls to action during the pandemic was one simple word, "Onward!" With that word, I knew my matter or concern was addressed and enough was said. The ball was in my court, and it was time for action.

David lives in Virginia but travels to Atlanta often for personal business and A.G. Rhodes board commitments. David started out as a board member under the leadership of his father, Rhodes Perdue, who led the organization through a period of great growth. He oversaw the organization's expansion in the 1990s when we went from operating one nursing home to operating three. When David took the reins, he furthered our impact in the community and all our homes added state-of-the-art rehabilitation gyms to increase our portfolio of services. Under his leadership, David has recruited an impressive cadre of Atlanta business and community leaders to join the board, including his sister—Margaret Perdue Denny—a career fundraising, and development professional.

David was in Atlanta in early March 2020, and I met him for lunch, along with the vice chair of the board, Jack Wilcox. We discussed several A.G. Rhodes matters but COVID-19 was chief among them. We had no cases yet, but we knew that it was only a matter of time. David and Jack wanted to know about the organization's preparation and how the board could be of more assistance to us. David left from Atlanta for a small family vacation, and while he was there, cases started to emerge rapidly in Atlanta nursing homes.

David and I spoke on the telephone while he was on vacation, and he decided to convene his executive committee the following day, Friday 13th (how ironic). The agenda for the call was similar to our conversation over lunch days earlier: how prepared were we and how can the board assist. This meeting turned into a standing weekly Friday morning call we held for several months then eventually occurred bi-weekly and then monthly. Time was wisely utilized during these calls. I would prepare a written report and e-mail it the night before so that our meetings were succinct but effective. We would not only discuss COVID-related issues but the many other business functions that had to continue regardless of COVID.

These calls, as well as daily conversations I had with trustees, formed an essential part of our crisis preparation. To feel as supported as I was made all the difference. I had the backing of the trustees which gave me confidence in my decisions. I wasn't encumbered by fear or paralysis, which can sometimes overrun leaders in crisis situations. The executive committee assured me that the company's financial reserves were available for critical needs, and they offered sound counsel and careful critique. Most of all, they showed prudent and effective governance at this critical time.

From the calls with the executive committee, David would update the rest of the board. We would also continue to have trustees' and advisors' meetings via Zoom, and our members seamlessly transitioned from supporting us in person to supporting us virtually.

Too often, leaders only see the importance of "managing down" or "managing sideways." They concentrate their efforts on ensuring that their subordinates and peers understand the organization's goals and mission. "Managing up" is often either neglected or not given the same importance. Managing up is the process by which staff become aligned with their leadership's expectations, and where they are not aligned, expectations can be adjusted. The critical role of the board during this crisis gave me the ability to seamlessly manage up, down, and sideways.

Having weekly calls, board meetings, and general board support ensured the board was updated about everything going on in the homes. I knew what our challenges were and felt comfortable transparently sharing them with our boards. This enabled us to better manage the crisis on so many different levels and it certainly built trust between our support team and our boards.

As our ambassadorial group, the board of advisors was accustomed to having many opportunities to visit the homes and volunteer for various activities and events, especially at holiday time. With help from Kim, the director of our volunteer program, advisors pivoted to supporting our residents and staff in new, creative ways. They sent pictures, letters, and birthday cards to residents and donated activity kits to aid in programming in the homes. One of our board members and former television anchor, Jocelyn Dorsey, hosted a monthly Zoom current affairs program for residents.

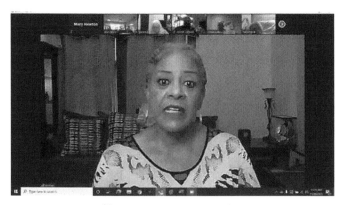

Zoom current events session

In July 2020, while still deep into COVID-19, our board of advisors changed leadership as it does every other July. Margaret Denny passed the gavel to Joni Towles, and without missing a beat, members continued to advocate for and support the homes in every way possible.

Keeping both boards informed was key to ensuring that our broader community understood our unique challenges and needs. If asked in the community about how COVID-19 was affecting our homes, members knew how to respond and they continued to develop the strategic relationships, partnerships, and engagement opportunities that benefitted us, especially at this critical time. Our boards took the approach of "It takes a village," and this provided comfort and reassurance for our support team and those working in the homes.

One of the board of trustees' most significant initiatives was to form a committee to oversee equity and inclusion initiatives within the organization. With that also came concerted efforts to bring more racial diversity to our boards. This was an ongoing goal, and we saw incremental changes to board composition over the last several years, but the events of the summer of 2020 put this effort into sharper focus. David became very active in board recruitment, but our board of trustees was already at its full membership capacity as outlined in the bylaws. Weary of changing the bylaws and potentially overloading the governing body, one of our board members, Larry Minnix, requested to step down to allow the trustees to recruit more diversity.

Larry served on the A.G. Rhodes board of trustees for five years following his retirement as the president and CEO of LeadingAge, an association representing more than five thousand nonprofit aging services organizations. Prior to LeadingAge, Larry worked for Emory Healthcare for twenty-eight years, including serving as the former CEO of Emory's Wesley Woods senior living campus. Larry's decision to step down was one of the finest examples I've witnessed of strong leadership and governance at its best—a leader putting the organization's mission and direction over his own, and an altruistic demonstration of diligence and integrity to make A.G. Rhodes better. It also served as a demonstration to all our stakeholders including boards, families, staff, and community of how serious the organization takes issues of equity, diversity, and inclusion. Fortunately for A.G. Rhodes, Larry continues to share his considerable talents in a different role now as he joined the esteemed group of trustees emeritus.

There are varying views on the role a board should play in an organization. Many prefer smaller boards over large ones and take a "substance over size" approach. Some contend that in a crisis, an overly involved board can get in the way and that members should "back off" and let management do its work unobstructed. According to Board Source, a nonprofit organization which supports, trains, and educates nonprofit leaders, particularly in the social sector, "There is really no one-size-fits-all approach to board structure… A board can be too big just as it can be too small" (https://boardsource. org/fundamental-topics-of-nonprofit-board-service).

My experiences during COVID-19 have shown me the extremely critical role that a board can play in crises if roles and responsibilities are well defined by board leadership. It has also shown me the importance of diversity of ideas and experiences among board members. Having individuals from varied fields and backgrounds ensures that members will help further the mission by providing meaningful contributions and counsel to leadership and staff.

Perhaps the best exemplification of this came after David and I visited the frontlines in late February 2021. We had a window of opportunity where we had no active COVID-19 cases, so the time was right, and he made a trip to Atlanta like a good general to visit his troops. We travelled together to each of our nursing homes, which David had not visited in a year. Although he and the rest of the executive committee heard from me weekly about the challenges that this crisis posed at each home, visiting in person was much different. After his visit, David sent the following e-mail to the rest of the boards and the support team.

To: The Board of Trustees; The Board of Advisors; Senior Support Team Members; and Administrators
From: David Perdue, Chairman Board of Trustees
Subject: Our Amazing A.G. Rhodes Team

Friends:

This past Friday I took the opportunity to pay a visit to each of our homes and spend some time "on the ground" with each of the administrators. Deke planned the surprise visits and we masked up and dove in. Wow! All of us have been kept apprised via communications and the website of how difficult this has been for residents, staff, and families of nursing homes. What I came to better understand on Friday is the level of emotional and physical stress that our administrators and their teams have undergone. In normal times, operating a skilled nursing facility is challenging. The level of regulation, the staffing, and the care of residents and families are just a part of the job description. Now ramp all of that up to unprecedented levels and make it literally continue 24-7 for a year and we can begin to understand and appreciate what has been required of our amazing team during the last year of the COVID-19 pandemic. There is also an emotional element that I am not sure that any of us can appreciate, but I had a peek at it on Friday.

Truth and Transparency lead to Trust. AGR has embraced those words and concepts from day one of this pandemic. We, as a mission-driven nonprofit, have done our best to care for all of our team members throughout so that they, in turn, can care for our residents. I am genuinely proud of and moved by this team and the leadership as I know we all are. I told each of these administrators that we knew that our success as an organization begins on the ground and not at the top. As I wrote this, an image came to mind…Greg, Kristie, and Mel (along with all of the rest of our folks that carry the load) must feel a bit like *Atlas holding up the world!*

I look forward to seeing you all soon in person and please know how grateful I am for all you each do to further our worthy mission. I will say again…I know now, after the last year, that A.G. Rhodes is truly a THOUGHT LEADER in addition to being the best service provider.

David

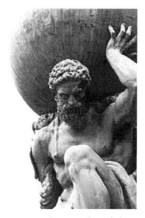

Atlas carrying the weight of the world

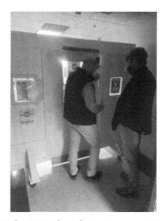

A.G. Rhodes Wesley Woods Administrator, Greg Heath, shows
A.G. Rhodes Board Chair, David Perdue, the isolation unit.

A.G. Rhodes Boards

Chapter 6

Double Pandemic

Guest Column appearing in McKnight's Senior Living on June 12, 2020:
We have always been essential

As a Black man who leads one of Atlanta's oldest and largest nonprofits comprised of a predominantly Black workforce, I join many others who are angry, hurt, sad, confused, and a whole range of other emotions concerning recent events across our nation.

I am deeply disturbed by the racism, injustice, and violence in a country where equality is promised and at a time when we should expect nothing less. I should not be scared for the safety and well-being of my family, my extended work family, or myself because we are Black.

The last couple of weeks have amplified the many complicated, systemic societal issues that must be unraveled and addressed before we can truly realize equality, and further racial divide will be detrimental to our progress. COVID-19 is clearly not our only crisis, and our industry—which has always stood firmly and strongly against ageism, ableism, and many other "isms"—must not be silent during this racism crisis. We cannot afford to be silent.

We must acknowledge that our direct care workforce is racially and ethnically diverse, but our senior leadership is not. We must be honest with ourselves and each other and have difficult and uncomfortable conversations that push us to change. We must listen and sympathize even if we don't have shared experiences, and most importantly, we must take steps to address the racial biases and prejudices which clearly exist. We must do more than issue statements. Words without actions are meaningless.

I'm proud to be one of the few Black leaders in this industry, but I'm even prouder to work alongside a compassionate, diverse workforce that has a more important role now than ever before. To the many others in this field who have been newly coined "essential" in our battle against COVID-19: It doesn't take a crisis for you to be essential. You—we—have always been essential.

As if COVID-19 were not enough. During the summer of 2020, we experienced what I call a "double pandemic." In addition to the challenges of COVID-19, the societal ills of discrimination and racism reared their ugly heads. While Atlanta should be a global epicenter for civil rights and equity, it was the just the opposite, and we became the epicenter for protest and petition. Atlanta is the birthplace of the civil rights movement and so many of its most ardent leaders, most notably Dr. Martin Luther King Jr. However, the reality is that we are perennially rated among US cities with the largest income inequality gap. In 2020, we ranked worst in the nation.

My guest column was inspired by the events that summer, especially because they hit so close to home. As a Black man, I was hurt and confused. It was a time of deep reflection for me. Many of our predominately Black staff were disillusioned. They looked to me for support, for solutions, and for action.

When the Black Lives Matters movement hit its peak during that summer, I was conflicted. To the passive observer, the organization I lead is diverse with a labor force of nearly 90 percent minorities—mostly Black—and me as a Black CEO. Many would not notice, however, that I was the only minority member of our senior management, and that despite a labor force comprised of mostly minorities, there was little minority representation in upper management positions. Most minorities are direct care staff and service staff, and this is not unique to just A.G. Rhodes. This demographic disparity exists in nursing homes nationwide.

I've had a few opportunities since becoming CEO in 2018—and when I was COO before that—to fill open senior management positions. Each time a position was open, there was no one who was a minority within the organization who I thought was prepared to make that step. In fact, no Person of Color had even applied internally. I had several external Black applicants, but I did not choose any of them to fill those critical roles. I began to question myself: Was I also guilty of the implicit bias that I so easily identified in others? Did I truly understand the plight of the African American, or was I looking at it through my cultural immigrant lens?

I grew up in Trinidad and Tobago—also known as "sweet T&T"—a beautiful twin island republic in the Southern Caribbean; the furthest island south to be exact. While Trinidad and Tobago has its own societal issues with race and diversity, many Black people run the government, businesses, and many other aspects of society. Because of my upbringing, I never felt like I had to prove anything to anybody. I wasn't a minority. I went to the best primary (elementary) and secondary (high) schools which were described as "prestigious." I also got an excellent university education, graduating with honors and as valedictorian of my undergraduate class. My parents and siblings were also brought up with great educational opportunities, and to a large extent, we were privileged and fortunate, which brought a level of confidence in whatever I did.

I migrated to the United States in 1999, got married, and had three children. While my children are still very fortunate in terms of upbringing and education, they are still Black and growing up in America. They have a much different world view than I did growing up. With the exception of two historic elections—one where we saw our first Black president, and twelve years later when we saw the first female and first Black and East Indian vice president—most authority figures, government, and business leaders do not look like them.

I always felt a great affinity for—and thought I understood—Black Americans. In particular, I've always been drawn to my staff and felt empathy for many of their life experiences. However, my wife Keya rightfully cautioned me about making judgements based on my upbringing or equating my life view and experiences with theirs.

Keya was born and raised in Brooklyn, New York, East Flatbush to be exact. She enjoyed a strong Caribbean cultural upbringing because of her parents and community, but she also sees the many biases and racist structures and systems created and perpetuated in the United States. Because of where I grew up, I was viewing the challenges facing Black Americans through my Trinidadian lens, which was not only unfair but led to incorrect assumptions. Even though I've experienced discrimination, I acknowledge that I have also made prejudicial decisions. This is something I have greatly worked on over the years, and before I pass judgement, I try to put myself in another's shoes. Although it's easier said than done, it's the only way to effect true change.

For most of us in the minority, there is an undercurrent of prejudice in just about every sector of society. We see it and experience it in the workplace and the marketplace. Most of us have been racially targeted at least once while running a mundane errand like grocery shopping. Most of us have been the subject of profiling and at times, intimidation by law enforcement. Most of us have been marginalized, sidelined, or disregarded at some point in the workplace. Even while I've been at A.G. Rhodes where I've had many wonderful opportunities to grow, I can still recall occasions where it was clear to me that race played a role in workplace decisions. I exude confidence because of my grateful history and culture, but it can be intimidating and lonely to be a minority in executive environments like boardrooms and industry leadership meetings. I am usually the only Black man, and because I'm an immigrant with a strong Trinidadian dialect, I sometimes have a level of nervousness about speaking. I take extra caution before I speak, and I'm concerned this may sometimes inhibit my best ideas and expression. I get more confident as I get more comfortable, but this is an unfortunate reality.

Most people cannot understand how years of this nervousness and self-doubt can take a toll on an individual. They do not realize it because they have never been in the minority. Being in the majority naturally brings confidence; some call this privilege. This is a conversation I have with my son all the time. He is a very good soccer player, but I see less talented players get recognized because they have a much higher level of confidence than he does. Thankfully as he gets older, he understands this more and he is determined to exude the same or more confidence, but it also means that he must work harder. The problem that many minorities face in the workplace is similar, having to work twice or three times as hard to be promoted or to get recognized in the same way as others.

The reality is that diversity in the workplace makes us all better. It can be the driver of positive organizational culture and enrichment. Different perspectives allow us to grow and promote innovation. We often assume that homogeneity is more comfortable, but that causes us to stagnate and fester. Without different life experiences, cultures, and backgrounds, our ideas and resulting work lack creativity. Only having one point of view doesn't reflect the true essence of the organization. Additionally, diversity is not only about race or sexual identity, it is far broader. Nationality, background, education, and skills are also elements of diversity. We need to hear and learn from all aspects of diversity to enable growth and improvement.

Quality providers practicing person-directed care openly speak out against ageism and ableism, but we also have a responsibility to our staff—to our essential workers—to ensure that discrimination and the other "ism"—racism—does not infiltrate our communities, whether it be implicit or not. As a promoter and practitioner of person-directed care and a strong vocal advocate of culture change for our industry, shouldn't I be as vocal about the many prejudices that affect my staff?

As a result of the double pandemic, I committed myself to parallel efforts. Just as I was determined to ensure that my organization was not crippled by COVID-19, I became equally determined to make a difference in the lives of our minority staff care partners. I advocated for our board to form the Equity and Inclusion committee to address areas where we lacked diversity. The board chair, David, was receptive and supportive. A few months later, when David suggested to me that we pursue a banking relationship with a local Black-owned bank, I knew that our committee was going to have true impact, and that I had the full backing of the organization's fiduciaries.

In its early phases and even while still fighting the pandemic, our committee oversaw several key accomplishments. The most meaningful to date is our Leadership Training Program, which stemmed from my disappointment that none of our minority staff—particularly Black staff—were qualified to fill previous senior management job openings. It was obvious that we needed to do a much better job at mentoring staff and helping prepare them for advancement opportunities within the organization.

This program, which was designed by me and my human resources director, Mary Helton, would provide leadership and mentorship opportunities and equip staff for potential management roles. Applicants of the program can choose one of two tracts: business management or clinical management. The program would give me and other senior managers the ability to mentor and maybe even sponsor well-deserving candidates.

The double pandemic profoundly impacted me. I shared my frustrations with many, and many of my White friends, colleagues, and acquaintances reached out to me, which gave me the opportunity to share my feelings. These conversations were educational for them, but they ended up being quite therapeutic for me to get all this "stuff" off my chest. One morning, I had one of these conversations with Mary Newton, my chief communications officer. Over the course of her eight years at A.G. Rhodes, Mary and I got to know each other well and she prepared most of my written speeches, articles, and presentations. Our normal preparation for these involved me sending her my thoughts or outline on what I wanted to say, and after a few back-and-forth edits and changes, the piece was ready.

I told Mary how I felt and that I wanted to write an editorial. Mary agreed it was a good idea, and we ended our conversation. I planned to start putting my thoughts into writing later that day but to my surprise, in less than an hour, Mary called me back and said she wanted to ask me a favor. Mary said she didn't want to be disrespectful, but she was touched by all I said, and as a White person, she never quite understood implicit racism as I had described it. The favor she asked was to take a stab at the first draft of the article based on what I expressed to her. I thought about it for a few seconds and said yes. The worse that could happen is that I wouldn't like it and I would politely make many edits. Mary was a very agreeable person and easy to be honest with, no chips on her shoulder! She also made it very easy for me by telling me, "Deke, if you don't like it, please let me know and I will understand."

The next day, Mary sent me her first draft and again included the disclaimer that she would understand if I didn't like what she wrote. The resulting piece begins this chapter and was published by *McKnight's Long Term Care News*. She nailed it! I sincerely appreciated her taking the effort, and to me, it was a sign that she understood— or at least tried to understand—how I really felt. It meant more than anything she could have said to me. Mary and I never really spoke much of this again, but I know that she was as appreciative of me allowing her to write it as I was appreciative with the result.

These heartfelt interactions are the only way that we can address our misconceptions, biases, and inequities as a nation. We need to truly listen to what each other has to say. The voices of the minority are critical, and we must understand that their perception is reality. Many of our words and actions, whether deliberate or not, have stigmatized and marginalized segments of our population. Only by directly addressing this through candid conversations and taking meaningful steps toward change will we come together as a society and finally begin to heal. The incidents of the summer of 2020 will forever be remembered as one of those watershed historical moments which defines who we are as a people. Let us hope and pray that our resulting actions will impact positive changes for years to come.

Chapter 7

Truth, Transparency, Trust

The three Ts: truth, transparency, and trust, are long-held principles of leadership, business, and public relations, and COVID-19 has highlighted their importance in our industry.

Nursing homes and other senior care providers have a long history of being heavily scrutinized. COVID-19 though put us under an even bigger spotlight, and we garnered more attention than ever before. That attention came from beyond our normal. Immediate stakeholders of residents, families, staff, and regulators, rather, we were thrust into the center stage of the pandemic and the public at large was watching us.

Early on during COVID-19, there was widespread doubt about the accuracy of reported cases and deaths in nursing homes. Among a plethora of data reporting requirements, nursing homes were required to report COVID-19 cases through the National Health Safety Network (NHSN) portal and via daily spreadsheet to their county's Department of Public Health (DPH). Providers in Georgia also had to report data to the Georgia Department of Community Health (DCH). There was a duplication of efforts as we were required to tediously enter the same data into many varying systems. These burdensome requirements took precious time away from resident care and led to increased risk of errors in reporting. The duplicative requirements also point to the disconnectedness of our local, state, and federal regulatory agencies: CMS, CDC, OSHA, FDA, OIG, DCH, DPH to name a few.

Whether deserved or not, there was a perception that nursing homes were hesitant to report COVID-19 cases and deaths. Death and dying are unfortunate realities in nursing home environments, and our staff must constantly face these realities in caring for a population as ours. The fact is that nursing homes care for seniors with many comorbidities and life-threatening illnesses. Each year, residents die from illnesses exacerbated by the flu or other ailments. Many providers were concerned that public reporting of COVID-19 cases and deaths due to COVID-19 would skew this reality. There were many theoretical conversations regarding true cause of death, and this likely contributed to the negative perception that some nursing homes were withholding key information concerning COVID-19 data.

Throughout the pandemic, and especially at the beginning, it was challenging—to say the least—to keep up with conflicting information from local, state, and federal leaders. It's not surprising that there was public mistrust as we had to continually change and adapt our approaches to meet ever-evolving information and ever-changing guidelines. While that's not something we could control or fix, we did—and still do—have some control over the public's perception of our industry.

When one is under so much scrutiny, a natural inclination might be to clam up. And this is very easy to happen. However, the only way the public will trust us is if we commit to truthfulness and transparency in everything we do—whether it be good or bad. Our reputations—and the reputation of our industry as a whole—depend on it. Trust me on this!

Unfortunately, because of this pandemic, the truth hurts! We care for the most vulnerable of populations. COVID-19 disproportionally impacted our senior population, and sadly, many of our nation's elders died. There's simply no sugarcoating it, and we shouldn't try to. We must be truthful about these harsh realities and the extraordinary challenges they bring. We must also be truthful about the ways in which we need to improve—or the help we need in order to improve—so that we can better manage the next crisis.

Being truthful, however, isn't enough. We must also be transparent. Transparency implies proactiveness in sharing information. As a heavily regulated industry, we're used to mandates that require us to share information, but we shouldn't wait for mandates to be told what and when to communicate. We need to anticipate questions, concerns, fears, and rumors and address them head on, and let our stakeholders hear it directly from us before they find out later through some other means. And trust me, the truth always comes out—your stakeholders will hear it through someone else if not from you. Further, when you're the source of your information, you're able to shape the message and interpret it for your stakeholders rather than leave it up for misinterpretation by someone else.

At A.G. Rhodes, we took a position of truthfulness and transparency in every aspect of our operations, particularly when reporting COVID-19 data. We reported more data than was required, and we explained the data so that stakeholders knew exactly what the numbers meant. At times, our data represented sad and difficult realities, but we had nothing to hide. We were being completely truthful.

We used our website as the hallmark of our transparent approach. We created a COVID-19 section that was constantly updated with resident and staff cases, deaths, graphs showing monthly trends, timelines, and very importantly, educational FAQs regarding COVID-19. Our COVID-19 web page was a true community resource which we could direct all stakeholders to. Families, staff, board members, the media, and others could use this page to access as up-to-date information as I had as CEO about the impact of COVID-19. Similarly, we utilized mass text messaging and e-mails to specifically keep families and staff informed every step of the way, and these communications would always point to the COVID-19 website section. This approach brought credibility to us as an organization.

Like most nonprofit organizations, A.G. Rhodes produces an annual report each year that we send to key stakeholders. This report summarizes our activities, events, and other operational highlights, and it details the organization's financial performance. The report has always been an example of our organization's transparency, but in our 2020 report, transparency was even more significant because of COVID-19.

It was not lost on us how much COVID-19 had consumed our lives and our operations. It was not lost on us that our stakeholders, more than anything else, were concerned about the residents in our care and the staff on the frontlines. It was not lost on us that we had an obligation to accept accountability for what was occurring in our homes while also trying to maintain our reputation in the community. It was not lost on us that the integrity of our organization would be put to the test more than it ever had before. We titled the report "Caring Through COVID," and it was illustrative of the organization's commitment to truth, transparency, and trust during these difficult times.

Even in times of crisis, commitment to truth and transparency will garner continued trust from your stakeholders to remain a viable and credible resource in the community. Because of COVID-19, our industry is facing another crisis related to our public image. The existing stigmas associated with nursing homes and senior care were exacerbated by COVID-19, and there is growing distrust from an already skeptical public. As we rebuild from COVID-19, our industry needs to adopt a more transparent approach to our operations. We should have nothing to hide, and we must ensure our stakeholders know that.

Chapter 8

Crisis Communications

Working in long-term care—and especially during my previous role as administrator—I have been through several crisis communications trainings. At a former company, I was even trained by a team of lawyers who were experts at managing crises through communications, and they began conducting annual training after one of the crisis incidents mentioned in the preface.

We run a tight communications ship at A.G. Rhodes, and crisis communications has always been an important component. My chief communications officer, Mary Newton, worked closely with me for the last eight years, well before I became CEO. Mary is top notch, an excellent communications professional. She's well versed in crisis communications with previous experience as a communications professional at the Federal Emergency Management Agency (FEMA) and as an air force veteran who served as a public affairs officer in various assignments including as a White House social aide. She exhibits all the professionalism you would expect from her military service and significant communications background.

Our external and internal communications efforts have evolved and improved over the last few years, which I believe gives us a significant advantage over many other providers that do not invest in communications. Not prioritizing communications is a big mistake. When Mary first started in 2013, I admit that I was skeptical—particularly of media relations and outreach—because our imperfect industry is highly scrutinized, particularly in the media. Proactive media relations and other communications outreach, even when positive, gave me pause. My colleagues and I quickly learned that this outreach was key to a strong communications program. Mary ensured we had a practical crisis communications plan that was updated annually. We also underwent significant media training. The media can be very intimidating, so we took the approach of getting staff accustomed to them early on to "break the ice." We also practiced speaking on camera, which is critical for media training.

For several years prior to COVID-19, we were used to the media and having them in our nursing homes. Generally, journalists were there to cover positive or feel-good stories regarding our residents and staff or for special events that garnered media interest. We often offered our organization as a resource when journalists needed a spokesperson from the nursing home industry, and over the years, we became more comfortable with media relations. In early March 2020, after COVID-19 emerged in the Washington State nursing home, we immediately convened a media training with key personnel. We correctly anticipated that we were in for turbulent times as an industry, and if we did not get in front of the message, others would craft it for us.

We trained organizational leaders for questions that they may be asked and prepared them for every scenario we could think of at the time. As CEO, I was considered the de facto spokesperson for the organization and many of our leaders assumed that in a crisis, the spokesperson responsibility would naturally fall to me. In a crisis, however, all employees of an organization are potential spokespeople and representatives of the organization. The possibility of a media "ambush" is always lurking. We knew that when some of the first COVID-19 cases in the United States were nursing home residents and staff, it was just a matter of time when it would appear in a Georgia nursing home and a matter of time before we became a target for media interest.

We received many media inquiries regarding COVID-19, and because of our crisis communications and media training preparedness, media outlets were often referred to us by our trade associations, the Georgia Health Care Association (GHCA) and LeadingAge. It was not unusual for a quote from or interview with A.G. Rhodes staff to be featured in the newspaper, television news broadcast, or industry magazine or periodical. Because of isolation and distancing requirements, we could not accommodate in-person interview requests so telephone, e-mail, and Zoom interviews became the norm. This took some getting used to as the experience was not as personable, and true feelings and emotion were sometimes harder to capture.

Media relations during crises like COVID-19 also provide much-needed opportunities to showcase positive things that are happening. For example, stories about the loosening of some visitation restrictions that allowed families and residents to finally reunite after months of separation or when staff were first vaccinated. These were opportunities for many providers to highlight "silver lining" stories, showcasing their efforts despite the difficult times. Proactive and responsive media relations can be double edged, however, particularly when bigger media outlets pick up stories related to your organization that result in a snowball of additional media requests from outlets that want to produce similar stories.

In January 2021, A.G. Rhodes was featured in an online national NBC article. This article garnered additional local and national media interest, and in February 2021, we were featured in a *CBS Sunday Morning* piece. The resulting notoriety led to more and more media requests, including interview requests with frontline staff. We decided to decline several interview requests because we did not want to take away staff's attention from their difficult work on the frontlines. We also wanted to respect the privacy of our staff and we didn't want to put them in potentially uncomfortable positions where their opinions or statements could be skewed or misinterpreted. While we understood the need to get our story out, we had to maintain the delicate balance between operating our homes, managing the public image of our organization, and maintaining positive media relations. It was a difficult balance even for the savviest of communications professionals.

When the seagulls follow the trawler, it is because they think sardines will be thrown into the sea. (Eric Cantona, France national footballer)

Like many nursing homes, we received our share of negative press. Nursing homes were the easiest target because we took care of the most vulnerable and the most at risk, resulting in the most impacted from COVID-19. It was easy for the press to publish negative stories about nursing homes as the numbers of cases rose steadily in our environments. Early on during the pandemic, we had to deal with a media outlet that attempted to correlate cases of COVID-19 with nursing homes that had previous citations on their annual regulatory surveys. Our Atlanta home, which only had four COVID-19 cases at the time, was named in the story because of a previous citation. Much deeper into the crisis when the Atlanta home had more cases, a family member gave an interview to a local television station, saying she was upset that her sister's roommate—and then her sister—contracted COVID-19. She also claimed that we were short staffed.

Our Wesley Woods home also received some negative press. In May 2020, a family member gave an interview to a local television station, suggesting that the facility should not take care of residents with COVID-19 and instead should transfer them to the hospital if they contracted the virus. Her mother unfortunately passed away in January 2021, and she again gave an interview claiming that her mother was unable to get the vaccine as scheduled because she had active COVID-19 infection.

Despite all that our staff were doing to protect residents and that so many factors were completely outside of our control, we were still vilified at times because these stories would imply a level of fault or negligence. With media relations, you must be prepared to take the bad with the good. You cannot welcome all good press and not expect occasional negative press. In all, I believe that media coverage of A.G. Rhodes was fair.

Frequent and proactive communication with families and staff was even more critical. We had been using e-mail communication with families for a few years, but in early March 2020—just in time for COVID-19—we implemented a mass text communication system to quickly send text messages to families. We used this to communicate regularly and openly during the crisis. Good news or bad, we let them know quickly.

If something was important enough to inform families about, then we also informed staff. Our employees are a key stakeholder. They can be our most positive advocates, but they can also be our most credible critics. We made sure they were informed every step of the way. Social media, video, e-mail, and other channels were useful in staff communication, and our two Marys, Mary Newton (communications) and Mary Helton (HR), worked together to ensure we sent consistent and well-tailored messages to staff through a variety of methods.

Among our staff, we have influential nontraditional leaders like long-serving CNAs, LPNs, or nurses. We know that these individuals—in many cases—are influencers among fellow staff, residents, and families. As a result, they are often perceived as more credible than managers or other leaders, and so we ensured they had the facts at their fingertips so they could help disseminate critical messages to stakeholders.

When I became CEO in February 2018, I made a commitment to staff to meet quarterly with them in the homes during informal town hall settings where they could share open and honest feedback with me about their concerns and issues. I also used these town halls as forums to update staff on the strategic direction of the organization and any other major organizational updates. These meetings continued through COVID-19, though now they were socially distanced. I would always tune into what the nontraditional leaders had to say, including their body language and facial expressions, as I spoke. Oftentimes, I would spend a few moments after to chat with them. They truly were in the know more than many of us in leadership could ever be.

Crisis communications can save a potential public relations nightmare. One does not need to be an Olivia Pope from the show *Scandal* to be effective at crisis communications. It should be viewed as a component of risk management. The more prepared you are and the earlier you appropriately act, the more likely you can mitigate significant risk and protect your organization's reputation.

One of the most critical resources in our crisis communications arsenal—especially during COVID-19—is our website, which was mentioned in the previous chapter, www.agrhodes.org. We created an online COVID-19 resources hub on our website that is not only a transparent library of COVID-19 data and frequent updates, but it also serves as an educational, credible resource. It links to CDC, CMS, and other regulatory bodies, thus verifying our protocols and policies.

A good communications officer will be able to anticipate issues, questions, and concerns and ensure that the organization is prepared to address them, but Mary would always remind us that we should never put the "cart before the horse" when it came to communications. Communications must go hand in hand with operations, but communications should not lead operations. In other words, you should never say you've done something, you're doing something, or you're going to do something without actually having the operational plans in place to do it. With this in mind, preparation is key, particularly in negative situations which almost always come with a crisis.

Staying well informed of what was happening operationally allowed us to stay ahead of concerns and this became critical, whether we were communicating about testing frequency, family visitations, outbreaks in the homes, vaccine hesitancy, or other updates. Our communication was honest, authentic, and timely, even when we didn't have all the information yet. Many of our COVID-related updates, for example, would inform stakeholders that more information was to follow as our next steps were still being planned or updated.

In early January 2021, Mary asked to meet with me in person and we met one Tuesday morning in my office. Teary eyed, Mary informed me that she was leaving A.G. Rhodes. She described this as the most difficult decision of her professional life. Mary was leaving to open her own communications consultancy firm. I accepted her resignation, and while I was very proud of and happy for her, I knew that her shoes would be difficult to fill. Mary truly brought a level of consistent excellence to her job. Without sound communications under her direction, I cannot imagine how we would have fared in this ultimate crisis of our lifetimes.

Chapter 9

Culture Change

The Nursing Home Reform Act passed in 1987 contained sweeping regulatory changes for nursing homes aimed at protecting residents and improving their quality of care. The act was a result of a 1986 study of nursing homes commissioned by Congress. The study, "Improving the Quality of Care in Nursing Homes," was published by the Institutes of Medicine and was critical of nursing homes, finding that abuse, neglect, and a substandard quality of care was prevalent.

The Culture Change Movement was said to have started in 1977 by the Live Oak Community in California *(Barkan, 2003)*, but the Nursing Home Reform Act was a regulatory impetus for organizations to implement meaningful reforms to existing practices. Despite this, and for more than three decades, culture change in nursing homes has been more of a theory than a reality. Regulatory oversight has pushed nursing homes to begin culture change practices, but care has still largely been based on a medical model characterized by staff productivity and industrial efficiency that contradicts many culture-change concepts.

In recent years, many providers have embraced culture change and have begun to focus care that accommodates the resident's individualized needs, wants, and expectations. Culture change addresses basic needs with a compassionate, practical approach that recognizes the human rights afforded to all of us regardless of age or diagnosis. Admittedly, the change process within our nation's 15,000-plus skilled nursing facilities has been slow and flawed. Nevertheless, the concept of culture change in nursing homes is indeed moving from theory to practice, and the outcomes prove this change is warranted.

In a culture of care, an individual's choices and self-determination are honored regardless of their medical condition or physical limitations. In this way, residents in nursing homes and other similar environments are given independence and dignity and afforded a great quality of life as they age.

Several organizations have emerged with the mission of assisting nursing homes and other senior living organizations to deinstitutionalize their practices through development of a culture of care that is considered person centered or person directed. The following table depicts the differences between a person-directed care model and the traditional nursing home model.

Person-Directed Care	Focus Area	Traditional Skilled Nursing Care
Focus on enhancing well-being of residents to reduce loneliness, helpless, and boredom.	**Overarching Philosophy**	Focus on operational efficiency and medical treatment for patients.
Care partners are encouraged to develop personal relationships with residents and participate in relationship-building activities such as sharing meals.	**Role of Staff**	Staff take a clinical approach to treating patients.
Family members are treated as care partners and are included in decision-making.	**Role of Family**	Family members are updated on resident treatment rather than being included in creating the care plan.

Nonmedical approaches are used to address resident behaviors, which are considered normal responses to the challenges of living with dementia rather than something to be medicated away.	**Responses to Behavior**	Medication is used to treat resident behaviors rather than trying to understand the root of the behaviors.
Residents can choose their own mealtimes and sleep schedules.	**Resident Schedules**	Residents follow set mealtime and sleep schedules that increase operational efficiency rather than meet resident needs and desires.
Facilities are designed to feel more residential and homelike.	**Environment**	Facilities feel more institutional rather than like a home.
Focus on on-site preparation of nutritious foods that respond to needs and desires of residents.	**Food and Meals**	Heavy use of processed or packaged foods and meals don't necessarily cater to individual needs.

The Eden Alternative® is one of the organizations that has assisted many providers, including A.G. Rhodes, along their culture change journeys. A.G. Rhodes' affiliation with the Eden Alternative® started in 2017 when the first of our three homes completed a significant milestone by being accepted to the Eden Registry, which is accomplished through an intensive and ongoing process where organizations demonstrate that they are changing traditional approaches to care by adopting person-directed principles and practices.

Since then, all three homes have earned Registry status, and we continue to learn, improve, and grow. Slowly but steadily, culture change is taking hold; it is a marathon not a sprint. It is a continuous process, and one that is gratifying and life changing on so many levels. It is wonderful to see the look on residents' faces as they appreciate and greatly benefit from our efforts. One of the most impactful moments I experienced was when a family member expressed to me how grateful she was for the way A.G. Rhodes cared for her late mom, and that it enabled her mom to live and die with dignity. Similarly, I am incredibly proud when I learn about the many staff who are asked to attend—and sometimes speak—at the funerals of residents whose loved ones were so appreciative of the care and love provided by staff.

Through person-directed care, we help residents continue to live a full and meaningful life just as we would want for our own lives as we age. We strive to provide a *Life Worth Living*, which is the title of an inspirational book by William "Bill" H. Thomas, M.D., a Harvard-trained physician, professor, entrepreneur, playwright, and performer. In his book, Dr. Thomas outlines how his experiences as a medical director in an upstate New York nursing home in the early 1990s sent him on a quest to implement a better and more humane way of caring for elders in nursing homes. He and his wife, Jude, founded the Eden Alternative® and established ten principles of care for providers that strive to help residents reconnect with the world and put the "home" back into nursing home. The Eden Alternative® presents an unconventional yet highly effective model of care and dignity which holds more relevance today than ever before (*Life Worth Living: How Someone You Love Can Still Enjoy Life in A Nursing Home,* William H. Thomas, M.D. VanderWyk & Burnham, 1996).

In 2018, I was asked to serve on the Eden Alternative® Board, which was one of the highlights of my career and one of my proudest achievements. As a board member and CEO that follows the Eden Alternative® principles, I have seen firsthand the difference in the quality of care locally and internationally among nursing homes that practice person-centered or person-directed care and those that don't. At A.G. Rhodes, I don't believe we could have survived COVID-19 without it. Our staff stepped up to act as surrogate family for our residents during a time when families couldn't physically visit their loved ones.

Families were shut out and limited from seeing the care given to their loved ones, and they needed assurance of utmost trust in the provider. Only bonds of trust with staff could give families the peace of mind that their loved ones were safe and that staff were doing all that they could to keep residents comfortable. Only these bonds could help families cope with the reality of the loneliness which they and their loved ones were experiencing. This trust between residents, staff, and families was truly tested, and nursing homes that did not see their roles as surrogate to the residents' families during these difficult months likely had more family complaints. They will experience challenges going forward in rebuilding trust and reputations.

I've been incredibly proud of our staff who have drawn on their Eden Alternative® education and training to help comfort residents who have been isolated and quarantined in their rooms. Our staff have been innovative, spontaneous, and compassionate. They have been family.

Stories from A.G. Rhodes Care Partners

Suze Berlanger, CNA, shared a message with families. She said, "I want them to know that we are the residents' family. They are my family. I know I'm not blood family, but we are family. I want them to know that we are trying to do the best we can for them."

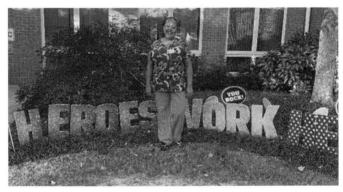

Suze Berlanger

Another care partner, *Fontella Favors, LPN,* stated, "People need us. This is not the time to be fearful, focus on the positives. Focus on what you can do to make somebody else's day and life better."

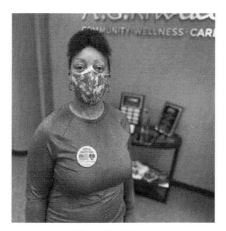

Fontella Favors

Rocquesha Ross, CNA, would pray with one resident who would tell her, "Pray this prayer with me, 'The Lord is my strength and my shield. I will trust him with all my heart.'" Rocquesha admitted she was afraid when COVID first hit, but her faith and trust in God eventually led her to volunteer to work in the COVID unit.

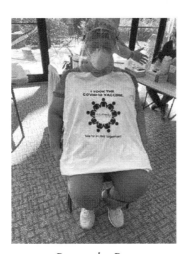

Rocquesha Ross

Overwhelmingly, our staff members express sentiments like these, and they selflessly and fearlessly put themselves on the front-lines every day not only to protect our residents' health, but to offer love and companionship.

Well before COVID-19 and as part of our person-directed care journey, we increased our usage of resident-friendly technologies that add more opportunities for robust and meaningful programming and activities. During COVID-19, these technologies kept residents connected to their loved ones through the isolation. The use of tablet computers for Skype and FaceTime calls helped immensely, and we relied more on mobile person-directed technologies including SimpleC resident companion devices and iN2L. These technologies have been in our homes for years, and in fact, in 2015, we were early adopters of iN2Ls mobile flex systems. We've even lovingly named these devices Wally and Jane. Jane was named after our chief development officer, Jane Simpson, who wrote the grant that funded its purchase.

Virtual family visit

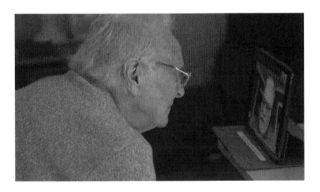

Innovation and technology also helped our signature programs, horticulture therapy and music therapy, adapt during COVID. Along with doing more one-on-one sessions, John Abel, director of music therapy, and Kirk Hines, director of horticultural therapy, produced videos that were played on the SimpleC Companions and on our in-house television channel.

To navigate the ebbs and flows of our COVID-19 outbreaks, music therapy treatments morphed from no live interaction during most of April 2020 to running small groups outside at all three communities when COVID-19 activity was low to conducting touchless music therapy from the hallways. During these sessions, John traveled the hallways, singing to or with each elder while standing in their doorway. Additionally, our Songs for Seniors program, which includes kits of mp3 players, headphones, and tailored music for residents, was able to continue seamlessly so that residents could access their own personal music on their own personal devices when they wanted.

Outdoor music therapy session

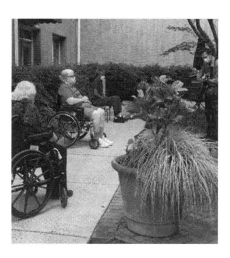

Kirk also adapted the horticulture therapy program as COVID cases rose and fell. When small, socially distanced group sessions weren't possible, he'd travel to residents' doorways and set up small stations for individual sessions with residents. He also ensured that resident rooms were adorned with beautiful plants and flowers and that arrangements and gardens outside—especially those in view of resident windows—were well pruned and beaming with life.

Horticultural therapy

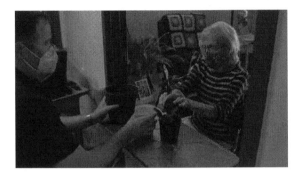

Bingo is a popular activity in most nursing homes. Many an administrator has unsuccessfully tried to change or adapt bingo to a more contemporary activity, all to no avail. Bingo is one of the residents' favorite means of socialization. Residents love the friendly competition of coming together, matching numbers, and marking their cards while waiting on the thrill and excitement of a resident loudly acclaiming, "Bingo!" This activity brought even more excitement at A.G. Rhodes as prizes were often the lure. Because of COVID, traditional bingo was adapted from a normally large group activity. Our activity staff quickly pivoted to offer an in-room version, with throw away bingo cards and chips. Numbers were called over the intercom system and residents checked cards in their rooms while staff walked the hallways waiting to hear the shouts of "Bingo!" before delivering winnings.

In-room Bingo

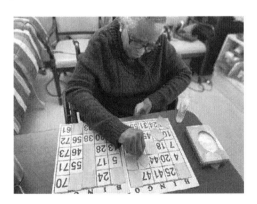

As with every facet of our operations, we had to remain flexible and adaptable with our programs and activities. Thankfully, much of the progress we made in incorporating more person-directed care practices throughout the three years prior to COVID-19 further proved to be significant and meaningful for residents' overall quality of life during the crisis.

The fact that we are still having conversations around culture change means that the pace of change has been too slow, and that is unacceptable. For many providers, COVID-19—the great accelerator—has relished and thrived due to a snail's pace of much needed change. Nursing homes that were not embracing change before COVID undoubtedly suffered even more than those providers who were on a path to improve care prior to the pandemic.

It is my desire that in years to come, we will not need to use labels or definitions for care like "person-directed" or "culture change." These should be natural expectations of care and to do otherwise is unacceptable. I also envision redefining what it means to age and to live in community. Labels and words like nursing home, facility, community, and so many others that are used interchangeably will not appeal to future generations living in our communities. Institutional care and treatment must be redefined to reflect the times and expectations and the emerging market.

Chapter 10

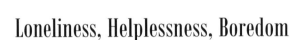

Loneliness, Helplessness, Boredom

On assuming office as the nineteenth surgeon general of the United States and to help inform upcoming priorities, Vivek H. Murthy, M.D., went on a listening tour across the country to speak to many Americans about their personal health and wellness concerns. In a book he authored that was published in March 2020, just before COVID hit, Dr. Murthy wrote, "One recurring topic was different. It wasn't a frontline complaint. It wasn't even identified directly as a health ailment. *Loneliness* ran like a dark thread through many of the more obvious issues that people brought to my attention, like addiction, violence, anxiety, and depression" (*Together,* Vivek H. Murthy, M.D., Harper Collins, 2020).

Francis Njuakom runs a charitable organization in Cameroon which focuses on vulnerable populations there. The organization Community Development Volunteers for Technical Assistance (CDVTA) fosters meaningful partnerships to positively affect the lives of the marginalized elderly in rural communities in Cameroon. CDVTA has impacted close to one million elders in their efforts to combat loneliness and encourage social inclusion and community solidarity with older adults.

Through strategic areas of intervention that benefit individuals and the society at large, CDVTA and Francis empower elders and help them provide for themselves in sustainable ways. Francis visits the United States yearly, invited by Jack York, Founder of IN2L technologies. Francis has also visited the residents at A.G. Rhodes. From my many conversations with him, it's clear that loneliness is not unique to the United States; rather, it's a worldwide phenomenon. In a way, loneliness can be regarded as its own pandemic that wreaks as much havoc as COVID-19. These two "pandemics" met in 2020 and the results were dramatic. Moreover, it exposed a painful reality that exists in our industry.

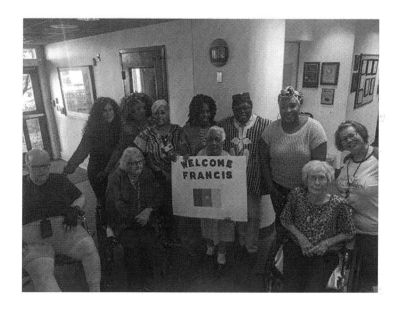

The physiological effects of loneliness have long been studied and have been directly linked to depression, substance abuse, and many other disorders and illnesses. If loneliness impacted many of us prior to COVID-19, all of us now likely cite it as one of the most salient consequences of the pandemic. Bob Kramer, founder and Fellow of Nexus Insights—a thought leadership platform that contributes to the transformation of housing and aging services for older adults—stated that one positive outcome from COVID-19 is that "It brought empathy to the issue of social isolation and loneliness in older adults."

Unfortunately, loneliness has always been commonplace in nursing homes. When Dr. Thomas founded the Eden Alternative®, his goal was to help eliminate feelings of what he called the "three plagues" common in nursing homes: loneliness, helplessness, and boredom. Now, there are ten Eden Alternative® principles which identify challenges and solutions for addressing these plagues and improving the well-being of elders living in nursing homes and other care settings.

> *Principle One: Loneliness, helplessness, and boredom are painful and destructive to our health and well-being.*
>
> *Principle Two: A caring, inclusive, and vibrant community enables all of us, regardless of age or ability, to experience well-being.*
>
> *Principle Three: We thrive when we have easy access to the companionship we desire. This is the antidote to loneliness.*
>
> *Principle Four: We thrive when we have purpose and the opportunity to give, as well as receive. This is the antidote to helplessness.*
>
> *Principle Five: We thrive when we have variety, spontaneity, and unexpected happenings in our lives. This is the antidote to boredom.*
>
> *Principle Six: Meaningless activity corrodes the human spirit. Meaning is unique to each of us and is essential to health and well-being.*
>
> *Principle Seven: We are more than our medical diagnoses. Medical treatment should support and empower us to experience a life worth living.*
>
> *Principle Eight: Decision making must involve those most impacted by the decision. Empowerment activates choice, autonomy, and influence.*
>
> *Principle Nine: Building a collaborative and resilient culture is a never-ending process. We need to keep learning, developing, and adapting.*

Principle Ten: Wise leadership is the key to meaningful and lasting change. For it, there can be no substitute.

In addition to the ten principles, in 2004, the Eden Alternative® identified seven domains of wellbeing to reflect the realities of those we serve as they age and experience health challenges. These domains are identity, connectedness, security, autonomy, meaning, growth, and joy.

Renowned geriatrician, author and colleague, G. Allen Power, M.D., depicts these domains similarly to Maslow's hierarchy of needs; however, he does not necessarily stress hierarchy, but instead emphasizes their suggested relationship to one another. For example, it's hard to create security without knowing someone well (identity) and having a consistent relationship (connectedness). Similarly, it's hard to achieve meaning and growth without security and autonomy.

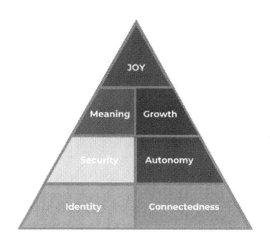

The Eden Alternative® Domains of Well-Being
Pyramid arrangement of domains by Dr. Al Power

Similarly, Sharecare Community's well-being index combines more than six hundred individual and social risk factors to measure well-being across people and places. Their individual health factors span five domains: purpose, physical, social, community, and financial. This is highly empirical research and analysis, and similarly points to well-being as the intersection of these domains.

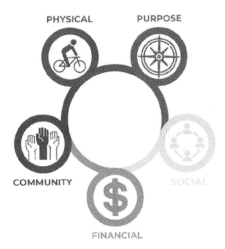

Sharecare Community's well-being index

In Dr. Thomas' book, *What Are Old People For? How Elders Will Save the World*, he wrote the following about well-being:

> Well-being is a much larger idea than quality of life or customer satisfaction. It is based on a holistic understanding of human needs and capacities. Well-being is elusive, highly subjective, and the most valuable of all human possessions. (*What Are Old People For? How Elders Will Save the World*, Author Bill Thomas, M.D., Vanderwyk & Burnham. Copyright 2004)

In Dr. Power's seminal book, *Dementia Beyond Disease: Enhancing Well-Being*, he questions the effectiveness of our current biomedical model of care in the nursing home environment and points to its damaging effects on the well-being of residents and staff alike. He powerfully and thought-provokingly challenges organizations such as ours that practice person-directed and person-centered care. He wrote:

> While many homes aspire to provide "person-centered care," the truth is that the departmental and organizational priorities nearly always trump the desires of the individual. One need only ask, "If an individual wants something that is inconvenient and requires some effort for the organization to accommodate, what is the likely outcome?" That is the true test of how person-centered we are, and few pass the exam. *(Dementia Beyond Disease, Enhancing Well-Being* [p. 104], G. Allen Power, M.D., FACP, Baltimore, M.D.: Health Professions Press, Inc. Copyright 2014)

Dr. Thomas's and Dr. Power's profound views on well-being resound for populations such as ours. Sadly, COVID-19 and the resulting restrictions threatened the well-being of so many of our vulnerable elders. Fear, isolation, restricted visitation, and stringent measures to protect residents did not promote well-being but instead were contrary to the principles and practices that we worked so hard to adopt throughout our person-directed care journey.

Robust social interaction, including meaningful events, activities, and an overall vibrant community, is one of the best indicators of a desirable nursing home and is a significant factor when one makes a choice on which nursing home to reside or place a loved one. One will usually get a sense—or a gut feeling—about the quality of a nursing home when touring one that either has or lacks a full social calendar for residents.

In her book, *Disrupting the Status Quo of Senior Living*, Jill Vitale-Aussem wrote about communities where interaction is encouraged, strong relationships exist between residents and team members, and staff and residents share communal spaces while interacting, including dining together. Unfortunately, even the best communities couldn't facilitate this type of environment during COVID-19. Staff couldn't provide spontaneous, interpersonal interactions, and families couldn't partake in the sense of community that they were so accustomed to.

At A.G. Rhodes, families have always been an integral part of our philosophy of care partnership and are very involved in the planning and delivery of care. As a critical part of the care partnership team, we often turn to family members for advice and assistance. They know the resident better than we ever could and can provide essential pieces of history, culture, or context regarding the resident which allows us to individualize care.

Prior to COVID-19, families at A.G. Rhodes would often volunteer; not only when it involved their loved ones, but also with other residents. Our best example is our *Jewels for Jewels* program. A family member, Arletta Brinson, whose mother was a resident at our Atlanta location, enlisted the services of her friends, church family, and sorority sisters to donate jewelry and other accessories for what became a treasure chest of items that would be distributed to residents in a jewelry-fair type event. Arletta's group would also host several culturally significant events at the nursing home, socializing as much with other residents as they did with Arletta's mother. Arletta continued hosting the program and volunteering even after her mother passed away. This is a pure, authentic example of care partnership.

During COVID-19 restrictions, Arletta still called us and lent her virtual support for our residents. She even adapted the popular Jewels for Jewels program by collecting donated items and dropping them off to be distributed by staff. Arletta said, "I have found a new family in all the residents at A.G. Rhodes. I do have some special 'aunts' who still call me, I share with them virtually and send 'love tokens.' The thing I miss most with COVID is my visits with them. A.G. Rhodes has given me the opportunity to give and receive unconditional love because of my volunteering."

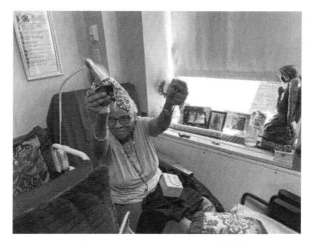

Jewels for Jewels adapted due to COVID-19

We must appreciate how well technology and other innovations were used during the pandemic to facilitate interactions among families, residents, and friends, and to keep the medical care of our seniors tantamount. But even though we can do a lot virtually, I have yet to see Zoom give tender loving care to an ailing resident. There are just some things that human interaction and touch are best for and cannot be replaced.

The lack of family and volunteer visitors has deeply impacted our vibrancy and the well-being of residents and staff. Probably the biggest public misnomer is that nursing home staff were relieved that families and visitors weren't allowed in our buildings during COVID-19. Nothing could be further from the truth. First, most nursing home staff appreciate the assistance given by families, visitors, and volunteers. Simple acts like a family member spending time with and observing their loved one, bringing them a drink of water or serving them a meal, gives a caregiver some respite during a usually hectic day. Second, we understand that we cannot replace the emotional bonds of blood relatives or lifelong friends. Third, most residents, especially those who may be agitated, anxious, or distressed, experience a sense of calm when their loved ones visit, and this effect may last well after a loved one leaves.

Holidays are normally the most vibrant time in our homes. During previous holiday seasons, our homes would host large, elaborate family dinners which were sometimes held over two days to accommodate the volume of family members who came to share a holiday meal with their loved ones. Hundreds of families and residents would attend, there would be music and performances from a live band, and a great time was had by all. This was one way we expressed thanks to our family members for entrusting A.G. Rhodes with the care of their loved ones. During the pandemic, we missed the buzz of families, volunteers, students, and others visiting, decorating, caroling, and simply spending time with residents. During the 2020 holiday season, we were instead overwhelmed by COVID-19 outbreaks, and our residents and staff missed many of the memorable activities and events that we were accustomed to.

Though we never took these festivities for granted, we gained a new perspective of their importance during the pandemic. Although we still prepared a holiday dinner for and celebrated with residents and we attempted to make it as festive as possible amidst our limitations, most residents ate in their rooms and participated in activities without the benefit of socialization with others. To make matters worse, two of our homes had significant COVID-19 outbreaks and had to implement even more stringent measures which further isolated residents. We tried our best during the 2020 holiday season, but it was not the same.

Our residents love opportunities to give. As an example, several years ago we began implementing more intergenerational programs and activities where our residents had opportunities to interact with and share important life lessons with youth. Through a summer program called Generation Connect, ninth and tenth-grade students came into our homes and participated in various activities interacting with residents. Students would interview residents about their past experiences, and they gained wisdom that can only come from residents sharing an emotional reservoir filled by a long life of events and encounters. The blessings of these exchanges were mutually beneficial as residents would marvel at the exuberance of their young counterparts and would inevitably draw comparisons with their own grandchildren, nieces, and nephews. Our Generation Connect program and these invaluable experiences were not possible during COVID-19.

Many of the measures and restrictions implemented during COVID-19 were driven by regulatory agencies and organizations.

For good reason, significant and stringent safety measures were put in place. However, the biggest contributor to loneliness, helplessness, and boredom during the pandemic was the social isolation caused by these health and safety requirements and the stringent visitation guidelines which the pandemic necessitated. Several families criticized us for following regulations or guidelines that they did not agree with. Regulations were intended to keep our residents safe and preserve life, however in many cases, I believe they had an adverse effect and instead hurt the well-being of our residents.

Our residents simply cannot thrive in environments where they miss those closest to them or are denied enjoyment from the bonds of friendships and interaction. We have lost easy access to companionship during COVID. Residents miss interacting with each other in activities, and staff miss interacting with residents and amongst each other. We miss going to lunch together, we miss hugging each other, and we miss feeling human again.

The domains of well-being are a telling depiction of what ultimately drives us. When the dust settles, the untold story of COVID-19 will be the many residents without COVID-19 who died from loneliness, isolated and unable to see their loved ones while feeling unsafe, afraid, and helpless. They felt their lives no longer had meaning. Sometimes we forget that people of all ages need to learn and grow. We assume that as people age, that desire diminishes. This is one of the great misnomers of aging. Joy does not have to—nor should it—ever diminish with age.

False assumptions about aging are dangerously rooted in ageist principles and practices, yet our current president was seventy-eight years old at inauguration. Our former president was elected at seventy years old and left office at seventy-four years old. Our nation's most respected infectious disease expert, Dr. Anthony Fauci, is eighty years old. Need I go any further? There is no correlation between age and growth. Our misguided assumptions about age and ability have led us to make decisions that are not in the best interest of our nursing home residents. Sadly, when outcomes are negative, we blame the nursing home and not the systems which have guided those decisions.

As we change the culture of our nursing homes, we need regulators to work with us in establishing common sense frameworks and guidelines that reflect and embrace the domains of well-being. These should inform a new Residents Bill of Rights that promotes a better quality of life and care. We know we must have sound regulations and guidelines to protect our residents' health and safety, but we must also have safe and careful plans that protect their well-being. There is a balance and as nursing home providers, we must show courage and stand up against regulations that infringe on the well-being of residents. We must use good judgement and act in good faith when caring for our nation's seniors.

After months of strict visitor restriction and restrictions to group activities, we welcomed regulations and guidelines that allowed us to offer more visitation and socialization opportunities. On March 10, 2021, CMS issued guidance which included the following excerpt:

> Since the beginning of the pandemic, the Centers for Medicare and Medicaid Services (CMS) has recognized that physical separation from family and other loved ones has taken a physical and emotional toll on residents and their families. Today, CMS is announcing guidance on expanding indoor visitation in nursing homes, in response to significant reductions in COVID-19 infections and transmission, resulting from ongoing infection control practices and high vaccination rates in the nursing home population following the authorization of COVID-19 vaccines by the US Food and Drug Administration (FDAs) authorization of COVID-19 vaccines for emergency use... Facilities should allow responsible indoor visitation at all times and for all residents, regardless of vaccination status of the resident or visitor, unless certain scenarios arise that would limit visitation... (https://www.cms.gov/newsroom/factsheets/cms-updates-nursing-home-guidance-revised-visitation-recommendations)

Late that evening, I received a text from Joan and Andy Immerman. Andy's mother, Rita Immerman, was a resident at our Wesley Woods home. Her ninety-fourth birthday marked the first day of COVID visitation restrictions on March 12, 2020. Her birthday festivities were cancelled just as the family reached the nursing home. After hearing the news about the relaxing of visitation guidelines nearly a year later, I received their text asking if they could come celebrate Rita's ninety-fifth birthday. They all received their vaccine and were hopeful they could hug their mom and talk to her without a plastic screen separating them. They explained that this was a special birthday and due to her condition, they did not know how many more they would have with her. I quickly responded that we would make it happen. On Friday, March 12, 2021, at 2:30 p.m., I was there to see the precious moment firsthand—mother, son, and daughter-in-law in full embrace. It was an extremely touching moment as Rita got the party she deserved. The rest of the family joined us virtually via Zoom. This felt right!

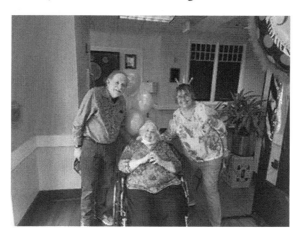

Now, as more residents, staff, families, and the general public are getting vaccinated, we are encouraged and hopeful that we can continue providing more of these essential opportunities. Our residents, staff, and families need them, and they deserve them.

Chapter 11

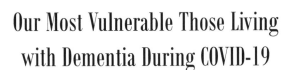

Our Most Vulnerable Those Living with Dementia During COVID-19

In April 2016, key board members and our most senior leadership gathered for a two-day retreat to inform our strategic plan—or as my predecessor Al would say, "Develop our road map." Representing the staff were Al as CEO, our chief operations officer, chief financial officer, chief development officer, chief communications officer and all three administrators. I was also there in a previous role—but new at the time—titled chief of strategic implementation. This role was created to usher the organization through a new model of care and other bold plans we had on the horizon.

While deep in strategic planning, our board chair, David, asked a seemingly simple question of the staff leadership. He asked who we thought were the most vulnerable of those we cared for. We unanimously agreed that the most vulnerable were residents living with dementia.

About half of our resident population is diagnosed with dementia or other cognitive illnesses, which is comparable to national statistics. According to the Alzheimer's Association, more than 40 percent of residents in nursing homes have some form of dementia and the CDC National Center for Health statistics estimates the number to be 47.8 percent. Although approximately half of our residents at A.G. Rhodes are diagnosed, we estimate that figure to be closer to

70–80 percent who are actually living with dementia. This estimation is common among nursing home providers, and some sources estimate that, "Up to two-thirds of all US nursing home residents have some type of cognitive impairment such as Alzheimer's disease" (https://www.ncbi.nlm.nih.gov/pmc/articles/PMC5767317/).

Many residents come into our care, and either before or while there, they develop signs and symptoms of dementia that are undiagnosed. Accurate and specific dementia diagnoses involve extensive neurological and other specialized testing and careful examination including a complete medical history. For various reasons, many do not undergo this testing either before or during their stay in a nursing home.

Dementia is an umbrella category of illness; it is not a specific disease. There are more specific diagnoses like Alzheimer's disease, Lewy-Body dementia, or Frontotemporal Dementia (FTD). Alzheimer's disease is the most common type of dementia. Although there are increasing numbers of early-onset Alzheimer's, the disease is still more commonly associated with aging and therefore nursing homes typically have higher rates than other care settings.

Most health care professionals in any realm of dementia care will agree that if you've seen one person with dementia, then you truly have only seen one person with dementia. Cookie cutter assumptions and approaches to dementia care are highly ineffective. Many living with dementia have been outspoken about these assumptions which they've stated are disrespectful on many levels. The fundamental beauty of the effectiveness of person-directed care is that it recognizes the individuality of each person based on their unique history, aspirations, skills, and abilities. While some basic interventions may work for individuals with similar histories, conditions, likes, and dislikes, in person-directed care we develop a more tailored plan of care as we learn more about an individual's unique needs and preferences.

The reality we acknowledged during our strategic planning retreat was that, although we identified those living with dementia as the most vulnerable group we cared for, most of our marketing efforts in recent years were focused on another group. We, like many other nursing home providers, were caught in a quagmire of prioritizing rehabilitation services in long-term care: physical therapy, occupational therapy, and speech therapy. These services were crucial to our survival and to stay in business.

While these therapies have positive outcomes for people living with dementia, individuals requiring short-term, subacute rehabilitation are more likely to access these services because of Medicare guidelines and higher reimbursements. Those insured by Medicare part A who require recovery after orthopedic procedures or after an accident or injury were the ideal nursing home patient from a financial standpoint. As a result, we, like most in the industry, developed a consumer model based on demand and reimbursement.

Most of our residents living with dementia require long-term care and their stay with us is covered by Medicaid, which does not fully pay for the services required for their care. We would subsidize their care with reimbursements received for short-term, subacute patient care. As a result, we tailored our marketing strategies to those individuals who needed short-term rehabilitation services and were covered by Medicare part A. This business model was a necessity for survival for most providers in the nursing home industry. At the height of Medicare reimbursement for these services, we even added "Health and Rehab" to our name.

Our board chair understood our difficult situation, but he challenged us in a way I will never forget. He told us that our approach was wrong and that our mission was to serve our community's most vulnerable. He challenged us to find a way to give more access to those who needed us most: those living with dementia and who had inadequate resources to pay for quality care. He told us that the board would make sure we had what we needed to stay true to our mission. Since then, our organization has been deliberate in our efforts to better care for those living with dementia. The strategic planning retreat changed the course of our organization and was the key impetus for our transformation to a person-directed model of care. In 2019, we even dropped the "Health and Rehab" from our name and added "Community, Wellness, Care" as our tagline.

Given that nursing home residents have been the most vulnerable during COVID-19 and that those living with dementia are our most vulnerable residents, it shouldn't surprise anyone that COVID-19 has had a devastating impact on nursing home residents living with dementia. We now have evidence, based on months of COVID-19 data, that the virus has had its biggest effect on those living with dementia in nursing homes.

Researchers from Case Western Reserve University in Cleveland, Ohio, analyzed electronic health records of 61.9 million people in America over the age of eighteen from February 1, 2020 to August 21, 2020. Their findings from that sample showed people with dementia had significantly increased risk of contracting COVID-19. Their research also showed that among patients with dementia, Blacks were twice as likely to be infected as Whites, pointing to serious health disparities among races (Wang Q. Q., Davis PB, Gurney ME, XU R. *"COVID-19 and Dementia; Analyses of Risk, Disparity, and Outcomes from Electronic Health Records in the US," Alzheimer's and Dementia. 2021; 1–10. https;//doi.org/10.1002/alz.12296).*

COVID -19 VULNERABILITY HEAT MAP:

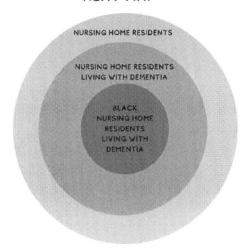

Heat map by Deke Cateau, February 2021

The heat map above is an illustration I created to highlight the severity of COVID-19s impact to the populations we serve. We experienced this firsthand at A.G. Rhodes. Many of our residents with dementia were difficult to isolate when outbreaks occurred and were most affected by the consequences of social isolation and other measures to stop the virus' spread. It was a virtually impossible task to keep residents living with dementia isolated in their rooms, and it was an enormous challenge for staff. It would stretch their skill and creativity to new limits.

Many of our residents living with dementia habitually walk from room to room and area to area, which is often referred to as a "wandering" behavior. Wandering causes concern for a resident's physical safety and the safety of other residents. Residents who wander will often take items that don't belong to them, which is often referred to as a "hoarding" behavior. Items such as silverware, cutlery, trinkets, condiments, and even clothing belonging to others are hoarded with surprising frequency. A cursory search of residents' rooms may result in an amazing inventory of objects and solve investigations into others' lost or missing items.

Wandering was even more challenging during COVID-19. Due to regulatory quarantine and isolation requirements, we frequently had to move residents from rooms that they were accustomed to and even lived for months or years. In many cases, we could not move furnishings, decorations, or other belongings which they were familiar with. Because of the frequency of moves and items had to be continuously disinfected, we simply could not bring them along for a temporary move.

It's important to note that when we use the word "behaviors" to refer to something like wandering or hoarding, we are referring to the physical manifestation of unmet needs for those living with dementia. For example, a resident who wanders may be trying to move or get exercise, and a resident who hoards may be struggling with sharing a room or may be trying to control or possess something they used to own and believes is still theirs. The risks of behaviors like wandering and hoarding were even more pronounced during COVID-19, and they contributed to the rapid spread of the virus.

(Read the Pioneer network, *"The Power of Language to Create Culture"* on *https://www.pioneernetwork.net/wp-content/uploads/2016/10/The-Power-of-Language-to-Create-Culture.pdf)*

When out of their rooms, mask-wearing compliance was virtually impossible for those living with dementia due to either the discomfort posed or because residents didn't comprehend the mask's necessity. Keeping masks on for long periods is a challenge for most of us, so how could we expect those with cognitive issues to comply? Emotionally, there were additional factors that affected those with dementia. Many residents understood that there was a pandemic, but many living with dementia could not cognitively interpret how that impacted them or the community where they resided. They couldn't understand how or why we were implementing certain measures. Additionally, the frequency at which we were required to make changes to comply with new guidelines made it even more challenging for them to understand.

To make matters worse, residents were now only seeing the eyes of their caregivers, which hindered their ability to recognize staff, read facial expressions, or see comforting smiles. It seemed sterile and impersonal. Mouths were covered with masks, shields covered faces, and bright-yellow or blue gowns covered clothing. How scary must this have been for our residents? Many no longer thrived. They were forced to stop walking, doors to rooms were closed, residents were quickly redirected back to their rooms if they tried to visit their friends down the hall, and many stopped eating. They deteriorated. When the administrator of our Atlanta home, Kristie, contracted COVID-19 and lost her sense of taste and smell, she said to me, "I don't know how our residents could survive this. Many of them already have diminished taste buds and now, they're all gone. That's why they aren't eating, Deke. That's why they're deteriorating." She was right!

There are many other clinical, neurological, and practical reasons why those living with dementia are more likely to contract viral infections, including COVID-19. Poor immune response and commonality of risk factors for both dementia and COVID-19 leave them more susceptible to contracting the virus.

A.G. Rhodes Wesley Woods is our only community with a unit dedicated to the care for those living with dementia. The secured unit is the entire second floor and can accommodate fifty residents. Since A.G. Rhodes Wesley Woods' first case emerged in April 2020, nearly all residents on the dementia unit—96 percent—have contracted COVID-19. Just two residents were spared from the virus. While our other two homes don't have designated COVID-19 units and instead operate an integrated model, well over half of those who contracted COVID-19 were living with dementia or some other cognitive illness.

Having a designated or distinct unit for those living with dementia is largely based on the realities of long-term care marketing and consumerism. The distinct and integrated models of dementia living are often seen as opposing points of view but are not necessarily so.

In Dr. Power's book, *Dementia Beyond Disease*, he strongly advocates for an integrated model as a more humane approach to quality of life and greater outcomes for all (*Dementia Beyond Disease*, Al Power. Health Professions Press 2014). Dr. John Zeisel, an internationally known expert on dementia care and treatment innovations, says a broad range of dementia care settings, including a distinct model, may be appropriate based on one's environment such as living at home or in a senior-care setting (*I'm Still Here*, Penguin/Avery 2013). He suggests a distinct model may be effective in secure models of care that are planned primarily for those living with cognitive disabilities. Dr. Power, on the other hand, argues with conviction that an integrated model in which all residents of all cognitive abilities live together increases the well-being of everyone along the continuum of cognitive health.

On face value, one may assume that the integrated model would make it more difficult to contain the spread of COVID-19, but in our homes, the spread was even greater in the distinct model. While there are multiple other factors that led to the spread of COVID-19, we must place significant thought and discussion on design elements related to those living with dementia as we restructure, rebuild, renovate, and improve. We need to balance quality of life with safety concerns, and we need to involve those living with dementia in these conversations to help inform our plans. We must stop at nothing to protect our most vulnerable, but this protection should not impinge on their quality of life.

Concerning statistics:

The number of people worldwide living with dementia is projected to reach 82 million by 2030 and 152 million by 2050 *(World Health Organization)*. The burden of Alzheimer's disease and related dementias in 2014 was 5 million people, which was 1.6 percent of the US population in 2014. This burden is projected to grow to 13.9 million in 2060, which would be 3.3 percent of the estimated population *(CDC)*.

This burden is even further and disproportionately segmented based on race and ethnicity. Among people aged sixty-five and older, African Americans have the highest prevalence of Alzheimer's disease and related dementias (13.8 percent), followed by Hispanics (12.2 percent), non-Hispanic Whites (10.3 percent), American Indian and Alaska Natives (9.1 percent), and Asian and Pacific Islanders (8.4 percent) *(CDC)*. Further, the rate of dementia is three times higher for people without a high school degree than for high school graduates (https://www.cdc.gov/media/releases/2018/p0920-alzheimers-burden-double-2060.html).

Over the last decade, we have seen a meteoric growth in "memory care" or "dementia care" communities where amenities and staff training are specifically geared toward those living with dementia. Many of these state-of-the-art communities have excelled in taking care of individuals with cognitive illnesses but most only accept private pay, which is simply not affordable for so many of our community's seniors. Thus, the underinsured, under resourced, and underserved cannot access these services, and this further adds to their vulnerability and risk for negative outcomes. As the great accelerator, this virus has not only accelerated great innovation and invention, but it has sadly accelerated the societal inequities of access to quality health care and social services supports.

One important lesson from this pandemic is that in the nursing home environment, any cookie cutter approach to caring for people living with dementia is inadequate and ineffective, regardless if residents are living in an integrated or distinct environment. The most up-to-date and forward-thinking approaches are those that prioritize respect for and dignity of each individual. They are person directed and aimed at improving the well-being for those living with dementia. Approaches, such as the Eden Alternative's® culture change approach and Dr. Zeisel's Hearthstone "I'm Still Here Hope and Engagement" approach, make great progress, but there is still more that can be accomplished, particularly as it relates to the unique needs of residents with different cultural and ethnic backgrounds.

Chapter 12

Testing

COVID-19 testing quickly became one of the most important weapons in our arsenal during the pandemic. In theory, if we knew who was positive, we could isolate them and stop the spread. However, there were many barriers we faced, including logistical, supply, and other challenges.

Three types of tests exist for detection of the COVID-19 virus:

Antigen testing, commonly referred to as rapid testing, seeks to detect protein fragments which are present with the coronavirus infection. These tests are typically conducted in a clinic or doctor's office or other Point of Care (POC) environment. Results are usually available within minutes. Positive antigen tests are usually highly accurate but false positives do occur. These tests also have a higher chance of producing false-negative results.

Polymerase Chain Reaction (PCR) testing seeks to detect the actual genetic material present within the SARS-CoV-2 virus infection. These tests are typically sent to a laboratory, which can take days to provide results. PCR tests have the highest COVID-testing accuracy and are considered the gold standard of testing.

Antibody testing tests blood for past infection by searching for antibodies present. These tests are also sent to a lab for results. Antibody tests are not normally used to detect current COVID-19 infection because it can take weeks for your body to make antibodies.

Both antigen and PCR test samples are obtained by using a nasopharyngeal or nasal swab, and later in the pandemic, a saliva test became available. Antibody testing is a blood test, so a blood sample must be collected.

Several COVID-19 tests received emergency authorization for use as community spread continued to grow rapidly. Initially, we contracted with local labs to use PCR tests. We began by testing residents who were symptomatic. This worked well for a few weeks as results came back within a day or two and enabled us to isolate residents quickly if they tested positive. Then more nursing homes began testing and labs struggled to keep up with the rapid increase. Results were taking several days to come back, which was problematic in our efforts to contain the spread. Additionally, we had an invisible elephant in the room: COVID-19 became notorious for the high percentage of asymptomatic carriers, and we began to see many of these cases, particularly with staff. We quickly adjusted our strategy to periodically test all staff and residents. As simple as this sounds, it posed many challenges.

I vividly recall in early April 2020 being on a conference call with my COO, Keith, the director of nursing at one of the homes and a staff member from the Department of Public Health (DPH). DPH offered to come onsite and conduct mass testing of the entire facility, including all residents and staff. While the idea sounded great in principle, we had a significant concern: What if a large number of staff results came back positive? How would we staff the facility if many employees had to leave and quarantine for two weeks? We asked DCH for some time to come up with an emergency staffing plan to account for this scenario.

Shortly after, states began deploying their national guard teams to conduct mass testing in nursing homes. Later in April, trained service members from the Georgia National Guard were deployed to conduct mass testing at A.G. Rhodes. Fortunately, the test results did not leave us with a staffing crisis. Even after the guard left, we started a trend of frequent mass testing throughout our homes. After all residents and staff were tested, we'd start the process again. Because results were often still delayed, we explored purchasing our own PCR machine.

After Keith and our clinical director, Jackie, conducted exhaustive research, we decided to purchase the Cephid GeneXpert system. This best-in-class machine eliminated the need to send PCR tests to a lab, and we could get results onsite quickly; two tests every forty-five minutes. This capability came at a high cost of $25,000 per machine and we required three; one at each home. These machines had the added advantage of being capable to give flu test results and a full respiratory panel of results for SARS-CoV-2, Influenza A, Influenza B, and Respiratory Syncytial Virus (RSV combination test).

There was a long back order on these PCR machines, but we joined the waiting list. In the meantime, we also purchased our own antigen test machines so that we could have some onsite testing capabilities, even if not as accurate. These machines were a fraction of the cost of the PCR machines; only $300. Clearly, you pay for accuracy. The antigen machines, BD Veritor Plus systems, arrived within a day, along with test strips which were in high demand. At about the same time we purchased the PCR and antigen machines, CMS announced a program to supply each nursing home in the country with an antigen test machine.

Along with a heightened focus on testing and to align with updated CDC recommendations, federal and state regulatory agencies released testing requirements which significantly increased our testing frequency. Frequency would be based on the county's positivity rate—the percentage of COVID tests that were positive—where the facility operated. If the rate was 0–5 percent, monthly testing of all staff was required; 5 to 10 percent necessitated weekly testing; and greater than 10 percent required biweekly testing. Although the requirement for resident testing wasn't as stringent, residents had to be tested weekly if there was an outbreak, which is defined as one or more cases. Resident outbreak testing would continue for fourteen days and restart if there were any new cases.

Taking a COVID-19 test is incredibly unpleasant. Nasopharyngeal swabs are the vast majority of what is used for both antigen and PCR tests and involves placing a long Q-tip-like swab through the nostril and down the nasal passage until resistance stops you from going further. The swab is then rotated for fifteen seconds to obtain a sample. This is an extremely uncomfortable procedure for everyone, including me. I have suffered from nosebleeds for years and the swabbing almost always causes me to bleed. I have now had the test many times, and each time, I ponder how this continuous invasive testing has become a normal reality of working in a nursing home. I also cringe that our fragile residents must endure such a test and how potentially dangerous it is to the staff administering it. Administering these tests increases the risk of infection through droplet transmission, and staff must be equipped with sufficient and appropriate PPE when testing.

In early September 2020, we tried using a saliva-based test to give some relief to our staff. We were encouraged that this would ease the physical discomfort of testing because for this test, one only spits into a collection receptacle. We purchased 350 kits per home to accommodate the volume of testing required. At $121 for each test kit, we spent $127,000 total. These tests had to be sent to labs, which were still overwhelmed by testing volume. Results again came back slowly, taking five days in most cases. This wasn't fast enough to be useful in mitigating spread. We quickly reverted to the nasopharyngeal antigen tests for our mass testing. Fortunately, the antigen test kits were much more economical, costing just over $30 each. Unfortunately, staff had to continue bearing the burden of a nasopharyngeal swab experience for up to two times weekly for the foreseeable future as the counties in which we operate all had high positivity rates.

Our PCR machines arrived in mid-October 2020, just in the nick of time as we suspected several false-positive results with the antigen machines. However, testing kits for the PCR machines were in high demand and thus supply was limited. We were provided three hundred tests per location with no guarantees for more until early 2021. We were quick to adapt and decided to use our limited PCR tests only as a confirmatory test for any antigen positive test results; a move that would ensure result validity and stop unnecessary quarantine. Ironically, while writing this book and just three months after our testing strategy was developed, the CDC updated information related to testing which resulted in updated guidance from our state and federal regulatory agencies requiring that all positive antigen tests be validated with a PCR test.

In addition to the obvious physical and mental strain posed to staff, testing also poses many logistical issues for nursing homes. Resident and staff testing continues to be one of our biggest challenges related to the pandemic. Other than the procedure itself, testing frequency requires that nursing homes keep up with the timing of the last COVID-19 case—also known as an outbreak—to ensure that there are no gaps in testing frequency. Additionally, the availability of testing supplies continues to be inconsistent. There are also many time-consuming administrative and reporting requirements as tests must be carefully logged and documented and positive tests must be reported to the DPH, DCH, and NHSN within a short time frame.

Contact tracing is perhaps the biggest challenge related to testing. The movements of those who test positive must be traced to determine if others may have been exposed to the virus, which begins a process to determine which residents and staff must be quarantined. During much of the pandemic, most residents were already restricted to their rooms, so contact tracing for residents who tested positive was a relatively simple process. Restricting many of our residents living with dementia and other cognitive illnesses, however, was not simple and significant spread occurred because of this. Contact tracing with staff was even more challenging.

Overall, contact tracing proved to be an important and effective process, and when successful, it undoubtedly minimized the spread of COVID-19 in our homes. Residents who tested positive were quarantined privately, and residents exposed to them were tested and also isolated or placed under observation. Even when a resident who was exposed tested negative, we had to account for an incubation period—time from exposure to development of systems—and there was always a risk the resident would eventually test positive. Staff who tested positive were to isolate at home for fourteen days (later changed to ten days) and could only return after that period if they no longer exhibited symptoms. After a resident or staff member tested positive, they did not have to be tested again for ninety days as it was assumed that they could not spread the infection for up to that period.

COVID testing has become a way of life for nursing home staff. Ironically, similar testing requirements are not required for many health care professionals who work in other medical settings that pose significant risk of contracting and spreading COVID-19, including those who work in hospitals. This seemingly double standard has contributed to a perception that nursing home staff are targeted and vilified. Regardless of perceptions, testing works. The more testing and the quicker the results, the better we can isolate, quarantine, and limit spread. Testing at some frequency is likely to be required in nursing homes for some time to come. One of the best investments we've made at A.G. Rhodes during COVID-19 is in our testing capabilities, most notably our PCR testing machines. The investment has not only helped us so far but will undoubtedly help us in the future.

Chapter 13

Vaccines: A Glimmer of Hope

Vaccines are one of the greatest health care innovations of all time and have stopped the spread of the world's deadliest and most infectious diseases. Before vaccines, millions of people died from the inability to control the spread of infectious diseases and because of this, CDC public health scientists list vaccines among the ten greatest public health achievements of modern times (CDC. *"Morbidity and Mortality Weekly Report,"* May 20, 2011).

Since the coronavirus pandemic began, the search for an effective vaccine was thought to be the best way for us to get back to some sort of normalcy. In that sense, a vaccine was a ray of light at the end of a dark tunnel. All credible sources said that finding a vaccine usually takes several years and in most cases, up to a decade. In the case of COVID-19, the federal government launched a program called "Operation Warp Speed" to expedite the development, clinical trials, emergency approval, distribution, and administration of the vaccine.

In mid-December 2020, we received word that two vaccines— one manufactured by Pfizer and one by Moderna—had tremendous success in the clinical trial phase and would be heading for emergency approval with efficacy rates of over 90 percent. Both vaccines were developed using messenger RNA (mRNA) technology. The vaccine was designed to give instructions to the body to make a fragment of spike protein of Sars-Cov-2. This protein causes the body's immune system to begin producing antibodies to fight off the infection, thus priming the body and protecting it against future infection. This technology is not new, and researchers had been studying it for decades with considerable success in vaccinating animals. This was the first time, however, that vaccines for humans had successfully been developed using mRNA technology.

In anticipation of a vaccine's arrival in October 2020, federal arrangements were secured with CVS and Walgreens pharmaceutical giants to set up onsite clinics at nursing homes and administer the vaccine. Both the Pfizer and Moderna vaccine passed the Federal Drug Administration (FDA) Emergency Use Authorization (EUA), and in late December 2020, distribution began with health care personnel and residents in long-term care facilities. Nursing home staff were prioritized to be among the first on a tiered list for phased distribution and administration of the vaccine.

The A.G. Rhodes homes were among the first nursing homes in Georgia to be selected to host these onsite vaccine clinics. Our Cobb home received its first doses of the Pfizer vaccine at a clinic on December 28, 2020. The following day, a clinic was held at our Wesley Woods location. Ironically, our Atlanta location—which had relatively few COVID-19 cases until a significant outbreak started there in December 2020—now had the most active cases in our organization, but their first vaccine clinic was set for January 7, 2021. I can only assume CVS set this date before Atlanta experienced its outbreak because many residents and staff would not be eligible to get their first dose on January 7 due to their recent COVID infections. Fortunately, CVS set up two more clinics at each home—each set twenty-one days apart—so that those who missed the first clinic still had an opportunity to become fully vaccinated at the following two clinics.

Because the Pfizer vaccine must be kept at minus seventy degrees Celsius before being thawed, that generally precluded most nursing homes from administering the vaccine themselves due to cold chain and storage limitations. Once thawed, the vaccine vials cannot be refrozen for reuse and therefore must be administered or discarded. Given this and the complicated distribution logistics, we considered ourselves very fortunate to receive the vaccine so quickly.

In preparing for the vaccine's arrival, and to our disappointment, we learned a new phrase to add to our COVID vocabulary: vaccine hesitancy. Prior to the vaccine clinics, we distributed a short questionnaire to gauge resident and staff willingness to get the vaccine. Only 46 percent of staff who completed the questionnaire said they would get the vaccine, compared to 78 percent residents who indicated they would receive it.

There were various reasons for staff hesitancy. Approximately 90 percent of our staff are Black and given some historical and unethical misuse of vaccines and medicine in general with minority populations, some staff were distrustful. Several staff also had a history of allergic reactions and said they were worried about side effects. Others had religious exceptions. Many were distrustful of the emergency approval process and vaccines in general. Overwhelmingly though, the most cited reason for vaccine hesitancy was a perception that the vaccine was still too new and there was a lack of information about long-term side effects.

The rapid development of the vaccine meant that its long-term evaluation could only be seen in time. Its effects on pregnant women, for example, was unclear at the time the vaccine first became available. Our staff is comprised of 88 percent women and of those, 40 percent are between eighteen to forty-five years old. Some worried about the vaccine's impact on fertility. It didn't help that prior to the vaccine's approval, many credible scientists, physicians, and the media consistently reported that finding an effective vaccine may take years because of the rigorous quality control steps required to assure vaccine safety. There was a perception that even with abundance of resources that went into the vaccine's development, collaboration among the world's leading scientists and the rigorous standards the vaccine met to get an EUA, the speed at which the vaccine was developed simply didn't pass the smell test. To many, there were more questions than answers.

Another regrettable contributing factor to vaccine hesitancy was the abundance of misinformation readily available and promoted. We live in a time when false news seems to be overwhelmingly accepted by many. The lines between truths and untruths are blurred, even at the highest levels of society and government. This is exacerbated by the rapid transmission and acceptance of information—or misinformation—posted on the internet and social media. Erroneous vaccine conspiracy theories flooded the internet with claims like, "The vaccine alters your DNA, it'll give you COVID-19, it contains a microchip designed for government tracking and control!" These are just a few of the false narratives that were confidently reported by many and believed by even more.

At about the same time our vaccine clinics were underway, we began hearing more about new, mutated strains of the virus, and questions emerged about the vaccine's efficacy against these strains. All viruses mutate over time; this is nothing new. Many mutations go unnoticed, but some can make people sicker. Even in our yearly flu season, we are accustomed to constant mutations, and each year, an enhanced vaccine is available to help account for these mutations.

The new COVID strains were concerningly more transmissible, and around mid-January 2021, the media reported that the virus was spreading at an even faster pace. The two most popular strains that emerged were the B.1.1.7 and the B.1.351, commonly referred to as the UK strain and the South African strain. Both were geographically stigmatized after the countries where they were first identified, but both were now quickly spreading in the United States. The UK strain was said to be 50–70 percent more transmissible. Although the Pfizer vaccine was shown to be effective on this new strain, it laid seeds of doubt in the minds of staff. Likewise, the South African strain had so many unknowns because of its mutated novelty. The news now reported on the possibility of a third booster of protection for these new strains. Would we now have to get a third shot? Should staff wait on a vaccine that would combat the mutation? These questions undoubtedly led to further caution and hesitancy.

Because of our internal poll results and before the vaccine's arrival, we used social media and other channels to educate and promote the vaccine. I visited each home for social distanced town halls where I, along with the medical directors of our homes and our consultant epidemiologist, spoke to staff about the safety and efficacy of the vaccine and took questions. We also encouraged and promoted the vaccine in other ways including awarding free points through our wellness program that could be redeemed for gift cards and other items for those receiving the vaccine. All vaccinated staff would get a special t-shirt to wear prominently to support the vaccine among their peers. Additionally, all those receiving the vaccine were entered into a drawing for a chance to receive giveaways including $500 bonuses, paid time off, television sets, and more.

Prior to the vaccine clinics, we had several logistical concerns regarding the consent forms that were required to be signed by families and legally responsible parties. We were given short turnaround times to get the forms signed, and because families couldn't enter our buildings to drop off forms, we made several return methods available, including a secure drop-off box outside each home. Aside from those challenges and some minor glitches on the first day of the clinics, all went as smooth as could be expected. What was disappointing, however, is that after all our many efforts to educate and encourage staff, only 48 percent opted to get the vaccine. This figure was almost exactly what our internal questionnaire predicted and essentially, our education and outreach efforts barely moved the needle. Our situation was consistent with vaccine hesitancy statistics nationwide in nursing homes, but still disheartening for us. On a more positive note, 80 percent of our residents were vaccinated at the CVS vaccine clinics.

Vaccine mandates are an alternative that some providers have turned to. While A.G. Rhodes has a mandatory flu vaccine policy, the COVID-19 vaccine presented a different set of circumstances that have kept us from making it mandatory. First, at the time of writing this book, the vaccine was still technically under emergency approval from the FDA. Second, we acknowledged that some of our staff's concerns regarding long-term effects should not be minimized and only time can reassure them of the vaccine's safety. Third, outside of the CVS clinic dates, we didn't know if our staff would have easy access to the vaccine.

There was a nationwide supply and distribution issue related to the vaccine, and if we mandated it, could we get our staff vaccinated outside of these clinics? What about new employees, how would they be vaccinated? We also were in a precarious staffing situation and worried that if we required the vaccine, we would lose staff who may turn to work for other companies that didn't have a mandate. Because of these reasons, our initial position was not to mandate vaccination. We would, however, continue to educate and encourage staff with the hopes that as the weeks passed, staff confidence would grow. Additionally, we also applied and were accepted to become a vaccination clinic so that once we have access to vaccine supplies, we can make vaccination onsite easy and readily available for staff and residents. If supplies allowed, we also wanted to make the vaccine available for families.

Vaccine hesitancy in nursing homes became another point of contention for many and another way to vilify nursing homes and nursing home staff. A local television news station aired a story highlighting A.G. Rhodes' creative ways of encouraging staff, creating a buzz of urgency and incentivizing vaccination. Some public comments on the story that was posted to the news station's Facebook page took us to task. Viewers criticized us, calling our efforts "bribes," and they criticized staff who chose not to get vaccinated. Just like there was a perception that nursing homes were at fault if they had COVID-19 cases, a perception emerged that we were also responsible for vaccine hesitancy.

In early February 2021, the CDC published a report titled "Vaccine Intent, Perceptions, and Reasons for Not Vaccinating Among Groups Prioritized for Early Vaccination." This report compared vaccination intent through surveys conducted from September to December 2020 and pointed to a high degree of hesitancy among people younger than sixty-five. Only half of those studied between ages eighteen to sixty-four reported they were likely to get the vaccine. Young adults, Blacks, adults living in non-metropolitan areas, adults with less educational attainment and income, and those without health insurance had the highest rates of hesitancy. Individuals over sixty-five conversely showed a 10 percent increase in intent to receive the vaccine during this period.

These two groups, eighteen to sixty-four years and those over sixty-five, directly mirror our two largest stakeholders. Our residents being in the over sixty-five group and our staff mostly in the eighteen to sixty-four group. These reports created a concerning narrative that most of our residents were willing to get the vaccine while many of the staff whose job was to protect residents were unwilling. Although vaccine hesitancy in the general community was likely similar to what we were experiencing in the nursing homes, there was a perception that our staff should know better and do better because we are caring for such a vulnerable population. It was no surprise that this quickly became an operational and public relations nightmare for the industry (https://www.cdc.gov/mmwr/volumes/70/wr/mm7006e3.htm).

Many of our staff were reluctant to be among the first to receive the vaccine given many unknowns still being discussed by experts, litigated in the media, and in the court of public opinion. Their hesitancy though was often seen as refusal, which did not help the situation. In interviews with National Public Radio (NPR) and Georgia Public Broadcasting (GPB), Dr. Kimberly Manning, a Black physician and professor at Emory School of Medicine, defended health care workers who have declined the vaccine, stating that many aren't necessarily refusing the vaccine indefinitely, but instead they are giving a "slow yes" to the vaccine (https://www.npr.org/sections/health-shots/2021/02/05/962835966/some-health-workers-say-theyre-not-refusing-the-vaccine-they-just-need-some-time).

Dr. Manning compared the insistence for health care workers to get the vaccine as that of a pushy used car salesman. This is exactly how many of my support team felt. We were going all out to persuade people to get the vaccine, sometimes quoting facts which we struggled to explain and had no firsthand knowledge of. We gave our own testimonials, we did everything in our power to cajole, and did all we could short of taking them for a test drive. I was relieved to see Dr. Manning's comments and it gave me great perspective and hope. Today I would refine her assessment to say that we had become new car salesmen. The vaccine was a new make and model that was only recently on the market, without a track record or the many years of reliability tests and consumer report data to guide us. We were initially giving our staff only two opportunities to buy this car and our sales pitch was, "Now or never!" Many staff told us that they would likely get the vaccine eventually, but they thought it was too early. They were uncomfortable being among the first to drive this car and wanted more assurance of its safety.

In looking back, I think we stratified and alienated groups throughout this crisis by using public shaming or personal bias to sway opinion. While I completely agree in the need and urgency for the safety measures put in place, our strategy in reaching individuals was wrong. We stratified the mask wearers from those who did not, those who wanted their children to go to school from those who wanted virtual learning, those who wanted to get tested from those who did not, and now we were doing the same with vaccines. My view was similar to Dr. Manning's. We should stop saying that people are refusing the vaccine, and instead acknowledge that for many, their hesitancy is "a slow yes."

Dr. Manning's assessment was validated in March 2021 when an Ohio-based software firm, OnShift, released results of a survey it conducted with employees of senior living providers. Based on a similar survey it conducted at the end of 2020, OnShift reported that there was a 94 percent increase in positive sentiment around vaccination, indicating that there was a growing acceptance of the vaccine as more time passed (https://skillednursingnews.com/2021/03/nursing-home-staff-willingness-to-take-vaccine-jumps-94-since-december/).

I received both doses of the vaccine. I did it publicly for all staff to see and openly spoke about my reasons for taking it. I spoke to the staff not as their CEO, but as one of them—a Black man and immigrant, a double minority. I told them about my decision process to receive the vaccine. I did my research, I consulted with physicians I knew and trusted, and I weighed the risks versus reward. The risk of taking the vaccine was that I may experience some side effects, although more evidence pointed away from this as the overwhelming majority of those vaccinated reported doing well. Alternatively, the risk of not getting vaccinated was the increased chance of contracting COVID-19. Given higher health risks associated with Black people who contract the virus, that risk meant serious illness and even the possibility of death. The reward of the vaccine, on the other hand, was the possibility of 95 percent immunity and doing my part to bring this crisis to an end. The choice was clear, and it brought with it a glimmer of hope.

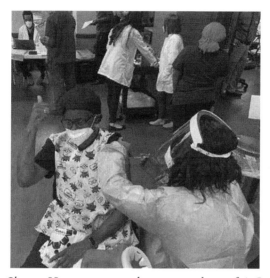

Sharon Hart, a twenty-plus year employee of A.G. Rhodes, was our first employee to get the vaccine

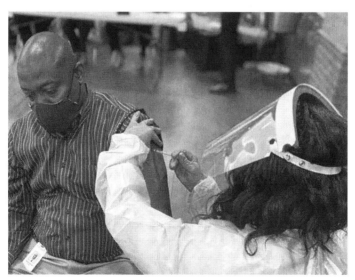

Deke Cateau receiving the vaccine

Chapter 14

Secret Sauce

Nursing home workers now have the most
dangerous jobs in America.

—*David Grabowski,*
Harvard professor and health policy expert

A.G. Rhodes has long held its staff up as our greatest resource. In an industry where we are taught that "The resident is always right" as a customer service mantra, it may seem taboo to admit that our staff is as important as any other stakeholder. At A.G. Rhodes, our philosophy is simple: If we take good care of our staff, then our staff will take good care of the residents. The Eden Alternative® articulates a similar golden rule: "As managers do unto the staff, so shall the staff do unto the elders."

The relational bonds between caregivers and residents have always been some of the most meaningful connections I have encountered. Staff demonstrate a nurturing spirit when caring for residents; it's as if they are caring for their own parents or grandparents. Forging bonds of trust become mutually rewarding for staff, residents, and family members who entrust us with the care of their loved ones. These bonds are cultivated daily by our staff, in particular our CNAs and LPNs. We firmly believe that our success at A.G. Rhodes is because of our staff.

For decades, we have built a strong and family-like staff culture. Everything from our benefits package to our management philosophies is meant to exemplify this. For example, our benefit packages are designed for every stage of our employees' lives, now and when they retire. Up until recently, we still offered a company-funded pension plan. When we transitioned to a more traditional tax-advantaged retirement plan, we did so at great cost in matching employee contributions.

Our company offered nine company-paid holidays, which is generous for our industry. Then after issues surrounding race and equity emerged in the summer of 2020, we added Freedom Day or Juneteenth as an additional paid holiday. We have scholarship programs for staff and even one for the children and grandchildren of our staff. We try to make our staff feel as appreciated as possible by demonstrating that we care for them beyond the walls of A.G. Rhodes. We care for their families, and we care for their futures. As a result, we have enjoyed great stability in staff tenure and relatively low turnover as compared to other providers in our industry.

Vickie Mathis was our longest tenured employee, serving forty-nine years at A.G. Rhodes until she recently retired. We have several more employees who currently work at A.G. Rhodes with more than forty years of service. Approximately 46 percent of our workforce has been with us over five years, 12 percent over twenty years, and our average staff tenure is 7.4 years. These are above average employment statistics in our industry.

In each of our homes, we proudly display our "Wall of Fame" which has a framed picture of each staff member in that community who has worked at A.G. Rhodes for twenty or more years. In our Atlanta home, the pictures have outgrown the wall and we had to add more wall space to display the staff's longevity. I often make the direct correlation between staff longevity, stability, and the quality of care we provide. Staff are the strongest indicator of good care and a good nursing home. They are our secret sauce!

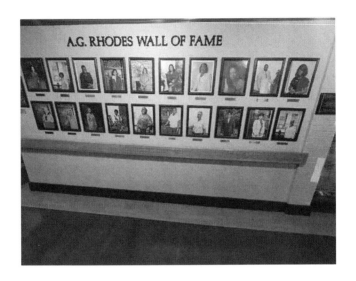

One of the most devastating consequences of COVID-19 has been its effects on our staff. While they have long lived with seeing the reality of illness and death in caring for a population as ours, nothing could have adequately prepared us for COVID-19. When we lost a longtime staff member over the summer of 2020 due to COVID-19, we were forced to face the cruel fact that our employees are just as much—or even more—at risk of contracting the virus. Nesteshia Harden, our coworker and friend, was just forty-six years old and her death had—and still has—a profound impact on us all.

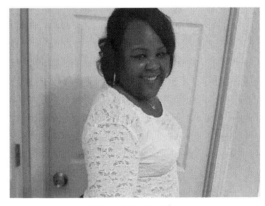

Nesteshia Harden

Staff were even more susceptible to contracting COVID-19 because our homes and their surrounding communities are in densely populated counties that—for much of the pandemic—had some of the highest positivity rates in the state. Staff live in these areas and no matter how careful they were, they could not avoid COVID-19 all around them. To make matters worse, because nursing homes had extremely limited visitation, it stood to reason that the main source of COVID spread throughout our buildings was our staff. The result was that staff were accused of not being careful enough, and they were once again vilified.

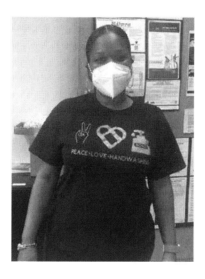

We encouraged staff to practice the sound safety precautions of social distancing, wearing masks, handwashing, and using hand sanitizer while at and away from the nursing home, but we had no way of enforcing it. When Nesteshia died, we became even more vocal with our pleas. At one of our homes, some staff wore shirts saying "Peace, Love, Handwashing" as another effort to encourage peers to follow important safety measures.

Park Springs, a local life plan community in Stone Mountain, Georgia, had staff voluntarily move into their community for eleven weeks. During that time, they did not return home to their families and lived together while caring for their residents. This was a truly heroic act, and while we explored the idea, it was impossible in our skilled nursing environments. In addition, our employees earn paychecks that are competitive in the industry but in some cases, less than adequate to support their families. As a result, many work multiple jobs to pay their bills. Those who work multiple jobs often work in another nursing home, which increases the likelihood the virus will be carried from one home to another.

The reality is that when COVID-19 cases increased in our surrounding communities, it was a matter of time before cases rose in our nursing homes, and the likelihood is that it was spread by staff. Others who were careful when away from work still faced the risk of contracting COVID-19 even when on a quick trip to the grocery store or from their co-workers or residents. It was a vicious cycle that fueled the spread within our facilities.

Recognizing the great risk to staff, we found additional ways to incentivize them for working in these conditions. Almost every nursing home provider offered COVID-19 "hazard pay" to staff agreeing to work with residents who had COVID-19. This came in the form of a differential payment or bonus in addition to their regular pay. At A.G. Rhodes, we took issue with this concept from the very start.

Admittedly, those working with residents who tested positive for COVID-19 were at greater risk, but the infectious and erratic nature of COVID-19's spread put all employees at significantly higher risk. For example, a staff member might care for a resident for weeks only to one day learn that the resident tested positive for the virus and was transferred to the COVID-19 unit. The employee would have obviously been exposed to the virus while caring for that resident and one could argue they were as much at risk as someone working directly on the COVID-19 unit.

We believed we needed to incentivize all for putting themselves at increased risk and we started a program in the homes called "Caring During COVID." We gave all staff a free meal each day; we gave periodic, significant bonuses to all staff; and in select months, we covered the employee's entire portion of their health insurance premium. We still paid a hazard differential to those working in the COVID units, but we felt all staff deserved additional compensation.

These incentives came at a significant cost to the organization and resulted in an average $3 per hour increase in staff pay.

We've maintained an unflinching commitment to staff during this pandemic, and it continues to this day. It reflects a century-long commitment from an organization that believes our mission should be equally as focused on our workforce. It is an "all in this together" family ethos of caring. More than anything else, we want our staff to know that we were there for them before and during COVID-19, and we will be there for them well after the pandemic.

As a result of the pandemic, our staff and others in health care have been newly coined as "essential," yet our workforce has always been essential. COVID-19 has been devastating in many ways, but we want staff to know that we are not a fair-weather organization, rather we are there for them in good times and in bad.

As COVID-19 improves in nursing homes, our industry must evaluate if we will continue prioritizing staff as our greatest resource through measures such as increased pay and benefits. For example, will we keep or take away the extra incentive pay that we have given staff for more than a year? How do we protect our essential labor force in the years to come? These are critical workforce questions that we must address.

Even prior to COVID-19, our industry has long suffered from high turnover rates and severe staff shortages due to high demand and limited workforce availability, particularly because we compete with hospitals and other settings that often offer more competitive benefits. Nursing home staffing issues have been exponentially exacerbated because of COVID-19, and my biggest concern is the future appeal of our industry to potential employees.

It will take years to assess the true impact of COVID-19 on our workforce, but it's clear that the consequences will be great. Without adequate pay and benefits, and public understanding and appreciation for their critical role, I worry about attracting frontline workers like CNAs and LPNs. Additionally, I am deeply concerned about COVID-19s impact on recruiting and retaining industry leaders and potential leaders. Who will choose an industry filled with such demanding regulatory burdens, stress, and public scrutiny?

These burdens already cause some nursing home leaders and those with strong leadership potential to move to a seemingly less stressful environment such as assisted living, independent living, or other levels of senior living care and services. Some leave the field completely, deciding that the rigors of nursing home operations aren't worth the stress.

During this crisis, I would have many conversations with our administrators about this. The administrator at our Wesley Woods home, Greg, is our most seasoned administrator with almost thirty years' experience. Greg and I spoke about how we have never experienced anything like the stress of COVID, and we would question why we chose this profession. In the end, we remained more committed than ever to fulfill our calling to be leaders and continue fighting the battle. I wonder about others though, who are not as hopeful. I wonder about future generations of nursing home administrators and whether COVID-19 will forever dissuade them.

The administrators of our Atlanta and Cobb homes, Kristie and Melanie, have just as much industry experience as Greg but prior to COVID-19 were both relatively new in their roles as administrators. I worried about them most during this crisis, but they also expressed a strong commitment in their resolve and showed admirable courage. Our COO, administrators, and I shared a unique bond during this crisis. We all understood the unique challenges of nursing home leadership during such a difficult time, and we had each other's backs.

As business leaders, it's easy for us to be engrossed in our daily tasks and in targeting operational efficiency. We can sometimes put empathy on the back burner, but we must make the effort to show the compassion and understanding that our staff need. We must also take the time to recognize that even as leaders, we also need to be comforted and reassured. This crisis has tested us all, and we have all been severely impacted emotionally, direct care staff and leaders alike. I have seen grown men and women—health care professionals—brought to tears by all that is going on around us, and the feelings of helplessness in fighting this invisible enemy while ourselves being at risk. I must also admit that behind the closed doors of my office, in the solitude of my home, or in the embrace of my wife, I, too, have shed many a tear. But the courage of our staff has encouraged me and lifted me back up. COVID-19 has exposed our human frailty but has also taught us how to empathize and heal together.

Chapter 15

Out of the Ashes, Build Back Better

> Never let a good crisis go to waste.
> —*Sir Winston Churchill, former Prime*
> *Minister of the United Kingdom*

The challenges of COVID-19 have brought to the forefront necessary changes for our industry, and to ignore these would be negligent. COVID-19 has provided the catalyst for us to re-envision our future and build back better. This is a watershed moment in our history and one that needs to be seized.

According to CliftonLarsenAllen LLP (CLA), median occupancy for nursing homes nationwide has dropped from 85 percent in January 2020 to an all-time low of 69 percent in January 2021. The state of Georgia similarly dropped from 87.4 percent to 71.4 percent during this time. On the contrary, occupancy in Green House and household model nursing homes has held strong during COVID-19. Not surprisingly, Green Houses had significantly fewer cases of COVID-19 and deaths largely due to their design and model of care ("Nontraditional Small House Nursing Homes Have Fewer COVID-19 Cases and Deaths," JAMDA, January 2021. Zimmerman, Dumond-Stryker, Tandan, Preisser, Wretman, Howell, Ryan).

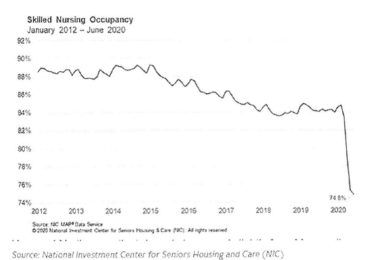

CMS Data and Green House/Small House Occupancy Percentage by Month

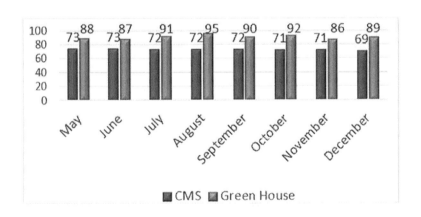

Will the dramatic decline in census for traditional nursing homes be a permanent trend which will require us to adjust our current business plans? It may seem quite plausible that many nursing homes will reduce expenses to accommodate for declining revenues due to lowered occupancy. Downsizing though may not be the answer because of high nursing home fixed costs like rents, mortgages, and utilities. Dilution of nursing home revenue streams has caused angst among nursing home providers, many of which are now on the financial brink. Even the nation's largest nursing home provider, Genesis HealthCare, in August 2020 expressed "substantial doubt" regarding its survival in the next twelve months.

Harvard professor, David Grabowski, points to this as the "fragility of nursing homes'" business model which has been "exposed by COVID." He calls for us to reimagine nursing homes and hopes to see more smaller settings like the Green House model and alternative payment models that will enable more financial stability (*McKnight's Long-Term Care News, "Big, Big Changes' Coming to Nursing Home Regulation Thanks to Pandemic's Destruction," Grabowski Says, November 16, 2020*).

Perhaps the solution is what Ryan Frederick, CEO of Smart Living 360, calls becoming, "Ambidextrous organizations…simultaneously exploiting today's business and exploring tomorrow's opportunities." As ambidextrous organizations, we would not abandon our traditional core businesses, but with increased vision and foresight, we would also consider exploratory business lines and growth through new product offerings. One may claim that some long-term care organizations are already doing this in mixed use models. Additionally, some providers already have complimentary lines of business in their portfolios including home health, hospice care, pharmacy, or other ancillary services. For these providers, decreased nursing home occupancy may lead to lower revenues, but they can help offset losses with increases in home-health business.

Ryan encourages us to dig even deeper and pursue disruptive innovation in our exploratory business. He postulates that the future of nursing home operations will be "a high risk and high reward game" (*Making Innovation Work, A Blueprint for the Seniors Housing & Care Industry*, Ryan Frederick. Point Forward Solutions, April 2015).

Larry Minnix, former President and CEO of LeadingAge and a member of the A.G. Rhodes board of trustees, has said for years that the nursing home industry is headed to a crossroads where only two types will remain: "The excellent and the nonexistent." In an interview with Dixon Hughes Goodman (DHG) Healthcare's *Southeast Finance Conference Magazine*, Larry also touched on high risk versus reward. He creatively used a card game metaphor to describe where we are as an industry and how we move forward. In Larry's "game," we are forced to play the best hand and organizations with certain characteristics have a distinct advantage in the game, including those with a strong culture and mission, those that have accumulated cash either through strong margins or fundraising, and those that have been able to create a true sense of community (*The 7th Annual Southeast Finance Conference, Looking beyond the pandemic, Volume II/Issue I,* January 27–28. Dixon Hughes Goodman).

Others claim that nursing homes will fade away and be replaced by home and community-based care and services. I believe our industry will shrink, but the demographic realities of an aging population will dictate that nursing homes will be around for quite some time. Our population growth for individuals over sixty-five continues to increase due to medical advances and wellness initiatives. The Silver Tsunami shows no signs of slowing, and by 2050, 20 percent of the US population will be over the age of sixty-five. These statistics resonate especially close to home because according to a 2016 *Forbes* magazine article, Atlanta is the most rapidly aging city in the US (https://www. forbes.com/pictures/edgl45hdlk/no-1-atlanta/?sh=71c659712bf0).

In the book, *The Longevity Economy, Unlocking the World's Fastest Growing, Most Misunderstood Market,* author Joseph Coughlin wrote, "Now that we have sketched the outlines of a new idea of old age, it's time to focus on how businesses can flesh out the picture" (p. 169). Products and services now have the opportunity and the market to respond. Consumers will expect no less. The greying of our society is guaranteed, and population aging is forcing us to prepare in so many ways that our nursing homes must either adapt or expire.

Home-based services are and should be our first option for senior care, but illness and disability create a true need for skilled nursing services. Dementia, too, continues to rise in our population, and proper care and services for those living with dementia is becoming even more difficult and costly to access. While the nursing home industry may compress due in large part because of the push to provide care at home, which has been accelerated by COVID-19, do not expect nursing homes to disappear. Expect them to get better. They will be fewer but more improved.

Assuming nursing homes will continue filling a critical community need, how do we come out of the ashes left in the wake of COVID-19? What is the course correction required to ensure that we are never faced with a crisis like this again and that our nation's nursing homes are sustainable for the foreseeable future? It is my contention that COVID-19 has provided the opportune moment for us to revisit our model of care, physical environment, regulatory framework, and business model.

Nearing the end of history's most destructive war, World War II in the mid-1940s, Sir Winston Churchill said, "Never let a good crisis go to waste." One can apply the significance of his words to what we're experiencing in our industry today. After all, many of our nation's greatest infrastructural and policy achievements occurred in the aftermath of a crisis, for example, the Great Depression. Infrastructure including 651,000 miles of roadways, 125,000 public buildings, 34,000 projects including airports, dams, schools, and hospitals were constructed. The Social Security Act, Fair Labor Standards Act, Federal Deposit Insurance Corporation, and the Securities and Exchange Commission all still exist today and are pillars of the American economy and society (*The Great Depression Top Five Public Works Projects of the New Deal,*" Bill Holland, February 24, 2017).

More recently, the financial crisis of 2007–2008 and the terrorist acts of September 11, 2001 led to critical system and policy overhauls of industry, which arguably serve us better today. Reconstruction in the aftermath of natural disasters like Hurricane Katrina is another example of our indomitable spirit in taking the opportunity to build back better. In this way, crises have led to significant improvements in our nation's critical infrastructure and policy.

So we must seize this opportunity to do likewise with the senior living industry and our nation's nursing homes. Several pressing opportunities exist, the four most pertinent are:

1. Regulatory reform
2. Increased wages for direct care workers

3. Improved financial model
4. Improved physical plants and environments

Regulatory reform

Nursing homes are already seeing increased surveys, audits, and regulations because of COVID-19, and we are likely to see much more in the coming months. An increase in the frequency and amount of punitive fines like Civil Monetary Penalties is almost assured. Some providers may exit the industry or decrease their skilled nursing services solely because of the more difficult regulatory and legal risk environment sure to increase post COVID-19. Invariably, these increases in regulation also increase paperwork and administrative burdens. This has a negative effect as paperwork becomes prioritized over resident care and adds expenses that should instead be allocated to direct care.

Most providers agree that the safety and dignified care of our nation's seniors is critical, and a strong and in-depth regulatory framework is required to protect our most vulnerable population. However, the biggest issues with current regulations are the enforcement measures. For regulations to be effective, enforcement must take into consideration regulatory intent and embrace a common-sense approach to outcomes.

I would predict that many substandard providers won't remain after profit margins have been withered away by the effects of COVID-19, and when the risk and liability involved in nursing home care comes to the forefront. A call for reform is not intended to excuse these substandard providers or make it easier for them to take shortcuts, rather reform should consider that most providers are doing everything they can to provide high quality care and services.

I advocate for a regulatory framework that is both instructive and educational and corrective at the same time. The need for penalties and other punitive measures for aberrant providers is necessary, but our system also needs to educate providers and work with them on best practices regarding caring for our nation's seniors. Our current nursing home regulatory system is only punitive, and we must put systems in place allowing state and federal surveyors to openly educate and document that education.

A system similar to the CMS Quality Improvement Program should exist in tandem with long-term care surveys to pivot inspections at high-performing homes into being an instructive quality improvement audit. This should become a hardwired part of the regulatory network. High achieving nursing homes should be rewarded and incentivized as much as poor quality ones should be punished.

Rather than react to the COVID-19 crisis with criticism, punishment, or cumbersome regulations that will only take away from the critical care our elders need, we need regulators and lawmakers to work together with providers to find creative solutions that better protect, support, and accommodate our elders and our staff.

Increased wages for direct care workers

COVID-19 has necessarily forced us as providers to take a much closer look at how we value our essential staff, and how we compensate our direct care workers. We don't like what we see. Much is now being published about the importance of paying a living wage to our care workers. One of the most comprehensive is LeadingAge's publication, "Making Care Work Pay," which makes a compelling case for the clear advantages of paying a living wage including return on investment through an increase in productivity and reduction in turnover and recruitment costs (Leading Age LTSS Center @UMass Boston. Weller, Almeida, Cohen, Stone. September 2020). Yet after so much discussion, we still have inequitable pay scales.

Over the 2020 holiday season, my twenty-year-old daughter got a job at a local retailer. Her starting wage was higher that most entry level CNAs are paid in this country. While I do not doubt how hard it is to work in the retail industry, I cannot help but see the inequity in our payment standards for nursing home staff who put themselves in harm's way daily, directly risking sickness and even death.

During COVID-19, providers had no choice but to pay hazard differentials to incentivize staff to work in such high-risk conditions. When stretched, we were forced to find a way to pay our staff what they deserved. Surely then we can get creative in finding ways to make these pay increases permanent. The fact that we even devote time to this discussion shows that we have a long way to go.

We operate our nursing homes with a hierarchical system of social classes where direct care and custodial staff are perceived to be blue collar and management staff are perceived to be white collar. We quickly identify and speak to the critical roles of our direct care and custodial staff, except when it comes to pay. We blame this on a broken system, but COVID-19 necessitates us all to take action, not individually or in silos, but as an industry. We should unify as one voice calling out on behalf of our precious human resource.

Payment models

Another strong catalyst for change in nursing homes that has been amplified by COVID-19 is our payment models and federal and state reimbursement patterns.

PPS: The Medicare Prospective Payment System (PPS) in nursing homes emerged from the Balanced Budget Act (BBA) of 1997. Under this system, nursing home Medicare payments are adjusted for acuity of services through a case mix system and also to account for geographic variations in costs. The result is a per-diem payment intended to cover all costs of services given to the resident including routine, ancillary, and capital related (https://www.cms.gov/Medicare/Medicare-Fee-for-Service-Payment/SNFPPS).

This fee-for-service program became highly lucrative for many providers because of its reliance on therapy services to increase the per-diem rate. In response to this, many nursing homes marketed themselves as therapy and rehabilitation centers and they even rebranded to reflect this. Volume of these services determined the payment more than the effectiveness of the services. This motivated all prudent nursing home providers to follow the trail of beneficial reimbursement patterns while providing quality care. Notably, many innovations have come out of this approach, including the upswing of subacute rehabilitation in skilled nursing settings. Subacute rehab has emerged as a method of choice for providers to supplement reimbursement gaps.

Transition to value-based reimbursements: In recent years, the federal government has recognized the need to transition to value-based programs where the quality and effectiveness of care and outcomes, more so than the volume of services, are key determinants in reimbursement. These systems typically incentivize and promote higher quality care and services and have been proven to be more cost-effective for a system already financially strained and nearing bankruptcy. In fact, in April 2020, just one month into the pandemic, the US Treasury 2020 Trustees Report estimated that the Medicare Hospital Trust Fund—the fund which finances Medicare part A payments—would be bankrupt by 2026. Approximately a year later and after significantly increased Medicare spending during the pandemic, estimates now predict bankruptcy by 2023.

The skilled nursing value-based program was launched in October 2018. This program uses hospital readmissions as a measurement to reward nursing homes with incentive-based payments based on the quality of care they provide to Medicare beneficiaries (https://www.cms.gov/Medicare/Quality-Initiatives-Patient-Assessment-Instruments/Value-Based-Programs).

Hospital policy trends have also greatly influenced movement toward more value-based programs. Hospitals remain the largest source of referrals for most nursing homes, and providers that monitor policy trends and use data to demonstrate quality and excellence are better positioned to get more referrals from hospital discharge planners than their competitors. This will be even more significant as hospital readmission rates and value-based programs determine the bottom line.

Effective October 1, 2019, the Patient Driven Payment Model (PDPM) was implemented. This system was the first major overhaul since PPS. It moves away from volume and toward value as a basis for reimbursement. This revised payment methodology addresses the overutilization of rehabilitation services and instead is based on a resident's specific clinical characteristics.

Several other value-based programs have been posited and tested as these types of reimbursement systems will most definitely form the basis of future payment models. For example, during the pandemic, a $523 million temporary value-based program based on COVID-19 infection rates and mortality was implemented.

ACOs: Accountable Care Organizations (ACOs) are groups of health care providers that voluntarily come together to administer coordinated, high-quality care to Medicare patients. ACOs receive a bundled payment for all providers involved, and when an ACO succeeds in delivering high quality care and spending health care dollars wisely, its participants share in Medicare program savings (https://www.cms.gov/Medicare/Medicare-Fee-for-Service-Payment/ACO). As of December 2019, there were 517 ACOs serving nearly seven hundred thousand nursing home residents as beneficiaries *(Inclusion of Nursing homes and Long-term residents in Medicare ACOs. NIH, Chiang-Hua Chang et al. Med Care, December 2019)*

Medicare Advantage: The rise of Medicare advantage plans and managed care organizations are also a trend that is sure to continue and proliferate the nursing home landscape. Medicare advantage plans, also known as Medicare replacement plans or Medicare part C, are plans approved by Medicare and generally follow Medicare rules. These plans are offered by private companies and, in essence, replace the beneficiary's Medicare benefits. By design, these plans also provide cost savings to the Medicare system and can have strict in-network benefits and in some cases, increased costs to the beneficiary.

Many of these plans have restrictive guidelines and have value-based programs and initiatives because they are the "payor" to the provider. An example is Medicare Special Needs Plan (SNPs) which restrict membership to individuals with certain diseases or clinical characteristics.

The astute nursing home provider would have familiarity and understanding of these plans as they are a significant alternative payment source and are proving to have large beneficiary enrolment. Forty percent of the total Medicare eligible population is currently enrolled in a Medicare advantage plan, and the Congressional Budget Office expects this to increase to 51 percent among the aging population by 2030. This trend is sure to create revenue cycle challenges for skilled nursing, however, providers need to become fluent in navigating the complexities of Medicare advantage programs as they are likely here to stay.

Medicaid: Medicaid offers state health insurance for elderly, low income, and people with disabilities. Medicaid is the largest source of payment for our nation's nursing home residents, however, in most states, this payment does not cover the full cost of caring for the resident. As such, a coverage gap is created, which nursing homes subsidize with other sources of payment. Medicaid has been a volatile source of payment for most states as its sheer volume challenges most state budgets. Medicaid has also been a national political volleyball as it is partially funded by a federal match which is controversial along party lines. Its perception as a welfare program is equally contentious, politically.

Because of its significant costs to states, Medicaid is also moving toward value-based alternatives in many jurisdictions, and in many states, it's operated on a managed care basis where managed care organizations oversee utilization and costs of the program.

The trend is clear: more value, less volume! Providers need to be prepared by ensuring improved quality, adding credence to Larry Minnix's claim that providers of the future will either be excellent or nonexistent. Should this hold true, we will see nursing home inventory reduction. The market will become less crowded, thus opening opportunities for innovation and creativity by those left standing that are committed to quality care.

Improved physical plants and environments

The National Investment Center for Seniors Housing & Care (NIC) estimates that more than 50 percent of the nation's nursing homes were built before 1980. Most are characterized by long hallways, large floors or units, communal dining, and activity areas, and of course, the abundance of shared occupancy. Of all the critical changes needed in our industry, this is perhaps the most daunting.

Most nursing homes have done a lot with very little resources over the years, and we have become particularly adept at "putting lipstick on a pig." But remodeling is no longer enough to bring nursing homes up to today's standards, however costs associated with replacing such a large percentage of this critical infrastructure will be astronomical. It has remained the elephant in the room in nursing home reform discussions for decades. How do we deal with this elephant? Former South African Bishop Desmond Tutu famously exclaimed, "There is only one way to eat an elephant: one bite at a time."

Being intimidated by, ignoring, or giving up on rebuilding efforts mean that we are abandoning critically needed infrastructural change, and in essence, we are abandoning the millions of lives that it will benefit. I take the position of if not now, then when?

The Green House model, which was founded by Eden Alternative® founder Bill Thomas, has successfully operated a viable and profitable nursing home model while affording high quality of life in an environment that allows well-being and purpose to its residents. This is a household model in which ten to twelve elders live together as a family, they have their own kitchen, living spaces, outdoor spaces, and residents live in private rooms. Other providers have built their own similar household model nursing homes with compelling environments for care. These models offer an attractive business case and the occupancy tables earlier in this chapter demonstrate how they have avoided the debilitating occupancy woes that most nursing homes faced due to COVID-19.

We need to approach nursing home design and construction differently than in years past. The institutional nature of nursing homes was originally based on hospital design and is no longer acceptable for today's seniors, let alone tomorrow's. Perhaps more importantly, today's nursing homes do not offer needed protection from highly infectious illness like COVID-19. Nursing homes should be built based on residential architecture and design to ensure that the experience in a nursing home actually feels like home and the environment is as safe as possible.

Traditional institutional nursing home architects should still be consulted to ensure that necessary life safety and building construction codes are adhered to, but the design elements should reflect a comfortable, homelike environment. They should have smaller living units or households, with living and dining spaces designed for smaller households. Single occupancy private rooms with private showers and baths should be available to each resident. Residents should also have easy access to therapeutic gardens and outdoor areas.

Another unfortunate omission from most current nursing homes are staff break rooms. Nursing homes were originally constructed for industrial-type efficiency which did not include rest, respite, or even a quiet place to eat and regenerate for staff. This is one of the most shameful legacies of our industry. In my twenty-plus years of nursing home experience, I have worked in or closely with nine traditional nursing homes and have visited countless others. None of them were built with a staff break room. Thankfully due to excellent and compassionate leadership, most of them were later retrofitted by repurposing an area or room into a staff break room.

To finance new nursing homes, I refer to so many of the major infrastructural projects across our nation, states, cities, and counties. We have an uncanny ability to get creative when it comes to funding schools, roads, parks, bridges, and other infrastructure needs. We can also look at examples of public-private construction ventures, such as those resulting in many of our sports teams' home stadiums and domes. Combined financing mechanisms provide significant return on investment for not only the private investor, but for our citizenry who accesses these services. These efforts also stimulate the economy through job creation from construction, and operation and revenue returns to state or municipal entities and investors.

I am not implying that owners and operators should not be responsible for new construction. New construction is a necessary cost of business and innovation. Properly done, it will lead to increased profits, so our free enterprise and market economy requires them to invest heavily toward this. However, because of current operating margins, owners and operators, even through venture capital investment, need financial support. Current nursing home ownership largely relies on real estate investment ownership and a tenancy model. This causes some of the high fixed costs that severely hinder revenue streams and can stifle innovative business models.

If current recessionary indicators continue and if we believe that stimulating the economy is the way to propel us back to stability, then there is no better industry to invest in than the long-term care industry, particularly nursing homes. Based on the success of the Hill Burton Act in 1954 that provided federal grants to stimulate nursing home construction, surely, we can get creative once again in our efforts to reimagine nursing homes for our future. While I am no financial expert, I know what can be achieved when the will of a nation is harnessed and coalesced, especially if it is done so on behalf of our elders.

Strategic reset: Emerging from the ashes will be more complicated than these four areas. I deliberately refer to these as opportunities because I believe they are attainable priorities based on industry trends and forecasts. These should be seen in both the contexts of our historical progression and maturity as an industry and us pursuing growth opportunities which create new value for our emerging customer base.

We are surrounded with lightening-paced change and innovation in virtually every industry and sector, and it should be no different in the nursing home industry. Through the current understanding of our business, we should have the confidence to be visionary in our approach to the future. For too long we have operated month to month, quarter to quarter, and year to year and must now widen our focus in planning.

Too many of our nursing homes have become "red ocean businesses," where we focus so intently on our competition and current trends that we begin to look like our competition and saturate the market (*Blue Ocean Strategy,* Kim Chan and Renee Mauborgne, Harvard Business Review 2004). We have been solely focused on operational effectiveness and have been so preoccupied with benchmarking to stay one step of our competitors in our skilled nursing pool that we simply start to look like them in whatever iteration is current.

According to Michael E. Porter, a professor at Harvard Business School, operational effectiveness is insufficient. The more bench-marking companies do, the more they look alike. The more that rivals outsource activities to third parties, often the same ones, the more generic those activities become. As rivals imitate one another's improvements in quality, cycle times, or supplier partnerships, strategies converge and competition become a series of races down identical paths that no one can win. Competition based on operational effectiveness alone is mutually destructive, leading to wars of attrition that can only be stopped by limiting competition ("What Is Strategy," *Harvard Business Review,* November–December 1996).

COVID-19s significant impact gives nursing home providers the perfect opportunity to do a strategic reset. The emphasis on culture change in nursing homes over the past thirty years demonstrates that providers can adapt their values, strategies, missions, visions, and a nursing home is both a business and a social service. Just as most companies' visions propel them to thrive well into the future, so too the successful skilled nursing enterprise must tactically approach the future with business foresight and intuitive planning.

Our management leadership and boards should engage in this process with intent and purpose. The process will often be uncomfortable, but discomfort is what usually brings innovation and change. COVID-19 has accelerated innovation and change in many industries, and ours epitomizes this well. While the nursing home industry is at a crossroads, we have seen significant advances over the last year in the acceptance of technology, innovation, and many of the critical path points which are needed to recover and rebuild. COVID-19 has also showcased the resilience of our industry. We have been through a barrage of attacks, and we are still recovering, yet we remain standing. Now we must focus on our future and chart a better way forward for our nation's nursing homes but, most importantly, for those who live there. Let us dare to dream as an industry; anything is possible.

As my board chair would say, onward!

Conclusion

*There is a reason why the rearview mirror is so small and
the windshield is so big, because where you are headed
is much more important than where you've been.*

I conclude this book as I began it. It is February 27, 2021, one
day short of a year since the first COVID-19 case emerged in a
Washington state nursing home. While COVID-19 is still very
much among us, the good news is that it has drastically declined in
nursing homes, which can be attributed to robust vaccination efforts.
Although slow to be distributed and administered and with notable
vaccine hesitancy among staff, the vaccine's effectiveness in providing
group immunity is clearly working.

Deaths in nursing homes are also following this promising
trend. With new cases in nursing homes dropping by as much as 80
percent and deaths by over 65 percent, the prioritization strategy for
the nation's most vulnerable is paying off. In fact, nursing homes,
which have been negatively targeted through much of this crisis, are
now serving as case studies providing evidence of vaccine efficacy
and herd protection. Vaccine effectiveness is also clearing a path to
reopening nursing homes to more families, volunteers, and visitors.

While we are much more hopeful in 2021 than in 2020, we cannot take our foot off the pedal. We must continue health and safety
precautions, or else complacency will become our greatest enemy.
Our staff though are exhausted. They are strained and desperate for
relief. Our brush fire has been smothered, but the right conditions
may easily bring it back ablaze. This current respite should not make

us overlook what has taken place over the last year. Although we have found an escape route, we cannot forget how this fire started.

When we finally do defeat COVID-19, we must not make the same errors of our past. COVID will likely not be our last pandemic, and its embers will be around for quite some time threatening to reignite and reinfect. We must use the time in between wisely. If history is to be a true teacher, then we must learn from the lessons of COVID-19. We must use the spotlight that our industry has been under to highlight every opportunity for progress and improvement. Never before have we been given such an opportunity, regretful though it may be, to harness the public support needed to truly make meaningful changes.

The popular quote at the beginning of this chapter is relevant to the nursing home industry, especially at this juncture. While we must never forget our past and have the obligation to use those lessons learned to help guide us, we should make no mistake that our focus must be on our future. Knowing where the potholes lay behind us is crucial, but more important is the understanding that even more potholes lie ahead. Avoiding those are critical for our industry's survival.

I hope that COVID-19 will be the catalyst needed for us to improve our industry. I hope we incorporate the leadership lessons we have learned over the last year. Not only lessons from the drastic impact of COVID-19, but also lessons of racism and social equity that permeate our nursing homes. I also hope that our perception of aging and treatment of our elders will drastically change.

COVID-19 disproportionately impacted nursing home residents and exposed many systemic and other issues which lay dormant for years but make no mistake that these issues are directly rooted in our society's view of our aging population. We place significant emphasis on everything that is youthful and young. Schools, children's hospitals, and just about any institution involving young people are prioritized, and sadly, we do not prioritize older adults.

In a conversation a few years ago with my development director, Jane, she compared how much easier her job was when she raised funds for childhood education compared to how difficult it is to raise money at A.G. Rhodes. Youth sells and old age does not. We see seniors as having lived their lives already, and today is for the present not the past. COVID-19 unearthed neglect not only for our elders, but for the systems and structures that are in place to care for them.

Writing this book has been extremely therapeutic for me. It has been the opportunity for me to express some of what I have mostly kept silent about for twenty years. Before COVID-19, I hesitated to express my views openly because I thought, *Who would listen and what would it do?* I, like so many, continued drudging along making the best of an imperfect situation and the cards we were dealt, and I used what tools we had to make every difference I could in the lives of the seniors in our care.

COVID-19 has inspired me to open up, and it is my sincere hope that these pages bring a greater appreciation for and understanding of the nursing home industry, particularly what we have faced during the pandemic. I hope it motivates others to work toward creating an environment allowing elders to thrive, not just survive.

I have learned in life that extremes create balance and promote change. There can be no true appreciation of heat without cold or sun without rain or good without bad. So let us use the negatives which COVID-19 has uncovered in our nursing homes to create the positive balance needed in our industry. And let us do this with a lens to the future. Let us rebuild thinking forward with intent and optimism. Let us create environments where we would all want to live in should illness or disability befall us. Let us look at aging with a progressive attitude toward transformation. We can and should dare to dream bigger and better.

"But when you give a feast, invite the poor, the crippled, the lame, the blind, and you will be blessed because they cannot repay you. For you will be repaid at the resurrection of the just" (Luke 14:12–14).

Acknowledgements

I give all thanks and praise to my Lord and Savior, Jesus Christ, for he has done so very much for me. All that I have is because of the goodness of the Lord and all that I am is by his grace.

I am blessed to have a loving wife, Keya, who supports me in all that I do. She has been my shoulder to lean on and my pillar during this difficult time. Our three lovely treasures—Danyel, Kiana, and Jeremiah—have served as my motivation, and without my wife and children, this project would not have been possible.

Other than the staff on the frontlines of this battle, I was also inspired by a group of angels to write this book: my grandparents, parents, and my parents-in-law were elders in their own right, and my brother's spirit continues to guide me. They are all deceased now but still lay watch over me. I miss you all immensely.

Lastly, I thank my entire support team and boards for giving me the honor of leading such a great organization.

About the Author

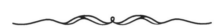

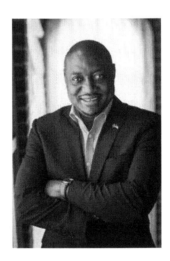

Deke Cateau is the chief executive officer at A.G. Rhodes, a non-profit organization providing therapy and rehabilitation services, short-term recovery, and long-term care at three metro Atlanta locations. Deke is responsible for a $45 million operating budget and approximately five hundred employees.

Deke has worked in the long-term care industry for more than twenty years. Prior to becoming the CEO, he served in various roles at A.G. Rhodes, including the chief operating officer, chief of strategic implementation, and he was the administrator for seven years at the organization's flagship location in Grant Park. Before working at A.G. Rhodes, Deke worked at Five Star Quality Care, Inc., a national senior living communities and services provider. He served in many capacities including area operations manager for Georgia, where he oversaw three skilled nursing facilities, eight assisted living facilities, and one continuing care retirement community. In addition to running nursing facilities in metro Atlanta, Deke has also managed a two-hundred-unit continuing care retirement community in Savannah.

As a leader in the fields of health care and aging, Deke educates the community—through robust outreach and speaking engagements with local, national, and international audiences—about the complex issues surrounding aging and long-term care. In 2021, the Georgia Health Care Association (GHCA) recognized Deke with its "Leadership in Public Confidence" award. In 2020, the Eden Alternative® recognized Deke with its "Tenacious Leader" award, and in 2019, Deke was awarded LeadingAge Georgia's "Award of Honor," which is the association's highest award presented to a distinguished individual who has provided outstanding leadership, exemplary service, and commitment to enhance the aging services field. In 2013 and 2014, Deke won the American College of Health Care Administrators Facility Leadership Award, and he won GHCA's Leadership Excellence Award in 2015. Deke has published two articles on long-term care: "Act as Though Your Customer is Right," Nursing Homes Magazine, May 2005; and "Skilled Nursing Facilities and Hospice Providers: Bridging the Gap," Nursing Homes Magazine, November 2006.

In addition to being a licensed nursing home administrator, Deke is certified by the National Council of Certified Dementia Practitioners as a certified dementia practitioner and a certified Alzheimer's disease and dementia care trainer. He is also a certified Eden Alternative® educator and certified Eden neighborhood guide, and a certified virtual dementia tour facilitator for nursing homes. Deke serves on the board of directors for several organizations including LeadingAge, LeadingAge Georgia, The Eden Alternative®, Georgia Health Care Association, and the I'm Still Here Foundation. Deke serves on several national stakeholder groups and committees, passionately sharing his knowledge and expertise in the areas of Aging, long-term care and dementia care. Deke is a Leadership Atlanta class of 2019 graduate.

Deke holds a bachelor's degree in history and a post-graduate diploma in international relations from the University of the West Indies, St. Augustine Campus where he graduated as valedictorian in 1997. He also holds a certification in Global Leadership Development from the University of the Virgin Islands.

Born in Trinidad and Tobago, Deke currently resides in Powder Springs, Georgia, with his wife, Keya, and their three children: Danyel, Kiana, and Jeremiah. When not working, Deke enjoys spending time with his family, cooking, soccer, and listening to Caribbean music.